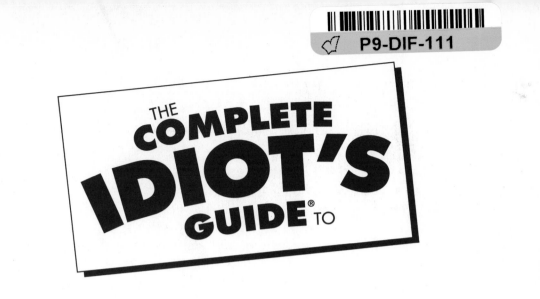

THE
COMPLETE
IDIOT'S
GUIDE® TO

Fighting Fatigue

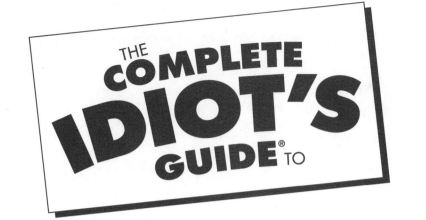

Fighting Fatigue

by Nadine Saubers, R.N., B.S.N.

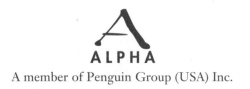

ALPHA

A member of Penguin Group (USA) Inc.

To my readers who I hope and pray have the same great outcome that I did in winning their fight.

ALPHA BOOKS

Published by the Penguin Group

Penguin Group (USA) Inc., 375 Hudson Street, New York, New York 10014, USA

Penguin Group (Canada), 90 Eglinton Avenue East, Suite 700, Toronto, Ontario M4P 2Y3, Canada (a division of Pearson Penguin Canada Inc.)

Penguin Books Ltd., 80 Strand, London WC2R 0RL, England

Penguin Ireland, 25 St. Stephen's Green, Dublin 2, Ireland (a division of Penguin Books Ltd.)

Penguin Group (Australia), 250 Camberwell Road, Camberwell, Victoria 3124, Australia (a division of Pearson Australia Group Pty. Ltd.)

Penguin Books India Pvt. Ltd., 11 Community Centre, Panchsheel Park, New Delhi—110 017, India

Penguin Group (NZ), 67 Apollo Drive, Rosedale, North Shore, Auckland 1311, New Zealand (a division of Pearson New Zealand Ltd.)

Penguin Books (South Africa) (Pty.) Ltd., 24 Sturdee Avenue, Rosebank, Johannesburg 2196, South Africa

Penguin Books Ltd., Registered Offices: 80 Strand, London WC2R 0RL, England

Copyright © 2008 Nadine Saubers

International Standard Book Number: 978-1-59257-773-6
Library of Congress Catalog Card Number: 2008920993

10 09 08   8 7 6 5 4 3 2 1

Interpretation of the printing code: The rightmost number of the first series of numbers is the year of the book's printing; the rightmost number of the second series of numbers is the number of the book's printing. For example, a printing code of 08-1 shows that the first printing occurred in 2008.

Printed in the United States of America

Note: This publication contains the opinions and ideas of its author. It is intended to provide helpful and informative material on the subject matter covered. It is sold with the understanding that the author and publisher are not engaged in rendering professional services in the book. If the reader requires personal assistance or advice, a competent professional should be consulted.

The author and publisher specifically disclaim any responsibility for any liability, loss, or risk, personal or otherwise, which is incurred as a consequence, directly or indirectly, of the use and application of any of the contents of this book.

Most Alpha books are available at special quantity discounts for bulk purchases for sales promotions, premiums, fundraising, or educational use. Special books, or book excerpts, can also be created to fit specific needs.

For details, write: Special Markets, Alpha Books, 375 Hudson Street, New York, NY 10014.

Publisher: *Marie Butler-Knight*
Editorial Director: *Mike Sanders*
Senior Managing Editor: *Billy Fields*
Senior Acquisitions Editor: *Paul Dinas*
Development Editor: *Ginny Bess Munroe*
Senior Production Editor: *Janette Lynn*
Copy Editor: *Megan Wade*

Cartoonist: *Richard King*
Cover Designer: *Bill Thomas*
Book Designers: *Trina Wurst*
Indexer: *Brad Herriman*
Layout: *Chad Dressler*
Proofreader: *Laura Caddell*

Contents at a Glance

Contents

Introduction

Despite the fact that fatigue is the most common complaint heard by doctors, it's still shrouded in mystery, uncertainty, and sometimes downright disbelief by many. Fatigue, like pain, is something that cannot be seen on a lab result, and so like pain it many times is classified as a "medically unexplained symptom." In other words, it has been implied by many and for too long that it just might be in your head!

Fatigue has the capability to deflate your tires—it can take the air out of every aspect of your life, including your confidence. And left untreated, it can become overwhelming and downright incapacitating.

Because more and more people are suffering with fatigue today, conditions that once were previously dismissed by medical doctors like Chronic Fatigue Syndrome (CFS), Chemical Sensitivity, Adrenal Fatigue, and Fibromyalgia are now accepted diagnoses.

Fatigue is the result of the cumulative effects of what I call *fatigue stressors* over time. Because it has many causes, it takes what they call in medicine a "multi-system approach" to treat. If you look at fatigue as a state in which all systems have been torn down by wear and tear, poisoned by toxins, and overworked to the point of exhaustion, you can understand that your plan needs to include building up with the right nourishment, resting while building endurance, and reducing your toxic load.

It takes time to reach a state of fatigue, and it also takes time to restore a state of health. So be patient with yourself and the process. No matter how severe your fatigue is, you can heal with time and commitment. One of the most important aspects of healing is believing it can happen.

How to Use This Book

This book will enable you to gain a better understanding of fatigue and learn its many causes. You'll also learn about the many options you have to help win your fight and finally how to put all the pieces together to make it work for you. I've organized the book into three parts:

Part 1, "Fatigue Facts," looks at what fatigue really is. It discusses certain fatiguing serious diseases and conditions and delves into the many other causes that might be working together or by themselves that result in or compound your fatigue.

Part 2, "Taking Charge of Your Fatigue," describes what steps to take first to begin the recovery process. It details your available medical options, the approaches and methods available outside of conventional medicine, and discusses different mental health practices that are available.

Part 3, "Taking Care of Yourself," helps you define your role and develop personal strategies that will give you the winning edge. Using the information in this part, you'll be able to create a plan to succeed based on the all the methods and techniques you've learned, along with your personal goals.

Extras

Throughout the book, you'll find a few aids that will help you along the way:

Energy Bar

Use these strategies to help combat everyday fatigue and help in your recovery.

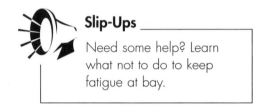

Slip-Ups

Need some help? Learn what not to do to keep fatigue at bay.

In The Know

It's never too late to learn. You'll find top-notch advice and words of wisdom from experts in the field.

def•i•ni•tion

These boxes will help you understand the meanings for terms and expressions you'll find within the book.

Acknowledgments

I'm deeply thankful to Pastor Robert Fuesler and to Carole Thompson whose support sent me on a trajectory course to success. I would also like to thank Jessica Talley and Jeseca Graves for their friendship. Both of them are shining stars, one here on earth and the other in heaven.

Finally, I'm grateful to John Davis and Nancy Deville for their ongoing support, which has made so many things possible.

Trademarks

All terms mentioned in this book that are known to be or are suspected of being trademarks or service marks have been appropriately capitalized. Alpha Books and Penguin Group (USA) Inc. cannot attest to the accuracy of this information. Use of a term in this book should not be regarded as affecting the validity of any trademark or service mark.

Part 1

Fatigue Facts

Even though fatigue is the most common complaint heard by doctors, it's still wildly misunderstood. Why is fatigue different from being tired or exhausted, and why does it affect so many people? To tackle this problem, you first need to look at the basics and understand the impact fatigue can have on your life. This part sheds light on how fatigue often feels worse than just being worn-out or run-down and reveals its many causes. You'll also learn how to identify behaviors, lifestyle habits, and other factors that can be fueling the beast.

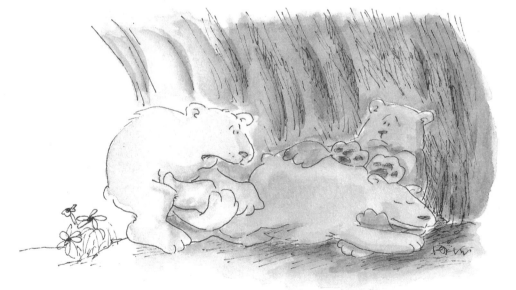

"C'mon, Helen! Enough already. It's May!"

The Rundown on Fatigue

In This Chapter

◆ Why fatigue is not just tired

◆ Understanding how fatigue costs you

◆ How does it feel?

◆ The domino effects of fatigue

After hearing just about everyone complain about fatigue in everyday life, its true meaning seems to have gotten somewhat watered-down. But the truth is fatigue, although its definition may be elusive to some, has far-reaching implications for your health and your life. Chances are you've had a hard time grasping exactly what is happening to you, but you might be coming to the realization that it's more than just feeling tired and run-down.

If fatigue were like a rash, everyone would be able to pinpoint when it first appeared. But fatigue is an insidious, unwanted guest that creeps in slowly, often masquerading as a symptom of just getting older. It tricks you for awhile until it begins to move in some of its evil cousins, like pain and depression. It could hang around for weeks or even months, deceiving you and telling you that it's only there because you didn't get enough sleep last night. But then you go on vacation or take some time off work and you are sleeping ten hours a night and you still don't feel rested. That's when it's hard to deny that something's wrong.

This chapter helps you better understand what fatigue is, how it can affect your life, and how you can recognize its many tagalong symptoms so you can start putting the pieces of your puzzle together. All through this book, we look at the gamut of mild to worst-case scenarios, such as Chronic Fatigue Syndrome. The reason is that therapies for the most severe also are used to treat mild fatigue and to keep it from getting worse.

Definition of Fatigue

So what exactly is fatigue? Fatigue is a sense of weariness, lethargy, and lack of physical energy that you wake up with every morning even after a good night's sleep. You have a decreased ability to function, a lessened efficiency in everything that you do, and a lassitude that is like an anchor you are dragging around.

Let's also get this straight so you know that your condition is not the same as your neighbor or friend who might quip, "You don't know fatigue, you haven't had my weekend!" Fatigue is not something you develop over a couple of days or something you can will yourself out of. You cannot "rally" as everyone seems to suggest, and you don't feel better if you just get out or go for a run, or anything else for that matter.

It's NOT Tired or Exhausted

Now let's get some other definitions straight. The true meaning of *tired* occurs when you don't get your eight hours of sleep or you toss and turn and don't sleep well. *Tired* is a normal response to lack of sleep, while *fatigue* greets you in the morning after a good amount of sleep. *Exhaustion* is the somewhat-expected result of working very hard mentally or physically. You can become exhausted after getting a good night's sleep followed by working very hard and, of course, it can be compounded by not getting adequate breaks, by stressors and demands, and by not getting nourishment and hydration along the way.

That's not to say you can't be fatigued, and tired, and exhausted at the same time, but for the purposes of this book and your understanding, remember those fundamental differences. You need to first understand that so you can see that fatigue, unlike being tired and exhausted, is not a healthy state. Fatigue is a red flag waving and a bugle blowing alerting you that something (or many things) is amiss.

Prevalence

First, because fatigue is a *subjective* condition, there isn't a lab test or x-ray that can be used to diagnose it. And, unless it's a true illness like it is with Chronic Fatigue Syndrome (CFS), it's really just a symptom. Fatigue, however, is both distressing and even disabling. Thus, people place high importance on it whereas doctors look at fatigue as a symptom of a vast array of medical conditions, an unhealthy lifestyle, stress, or a combination of these factors. Doctors start at the top of the list and consider the most common conditions that include the symptom of fatigue and begin to whittle down that list by looking at every possible cause in order to piece together the puzzle. Your fatigue is important to your doctor, but the cause is even more so!

def•i•ni•tion

Fatigue is a **subjective** symptom, which means it's not measurable by lab tests or physical exam. Like pain, fatigue is something that is described by the person experiencing it.

Because it is subjective and it occurs as a symptom of hundreds of different conditions, it's next to impossible to determine accurately how often it occurs in the population. So more or less, with estimates from many sources, we could guess that it occurs in about one in four people at any given time. Unfortunately, we do know that women experience fatigue twice as often as men do, but before you say it's because women's work is harder than men's work, we also know that fatigue does not correlate strongly with any occupation or even age.

Given that CFS is just beginning to gain acceptance as a "real" medical condition, again it is difficult to gauge its real prevalence. The Center for Disease Control has attempted to guesstimate and has come up with the figure of one million people in the United States who are diagnosed with CFS and tens of millions of people who have comparable fatiguing illnesses.

Fatigue Fallout

Just as a structure such as a bridge can become "fatigued" from overuse and misuse, so can your body. That structure doesn't become stronger after not being used for a week or a night—it's still fatigued. Unless you go in and correct the problems, chances are your body will fail and crumble. And like a failing structure, if you have stressed your body and mind to the point of fatigue, you need to address those stressors and

def•i•ni•tion

Fatigue has major impacts on your **quality of life,** or your ability to enjoy the activities of your daily life. Doctors frequently consider the effect that an illness or medical treatment has on your quality of life to determine such things as severity and risk versus benefit.

rebuild those weakened areas to recover fully and not crumble like a weakened and stressed bridge.

Fatigue is an enigmatic, cloak-and-dagger, and capricious symptom whose causes and characteristics are akin to layers of an onion that seriously impacts your *quality of life*. It can rob you of your dreams, steal your joy and passion, and deplete your bank account. Fatigue is like a ball rolling that is collecting debris and getting larger, more all-consuming, and destructive in your life as it progresses.

Health and Safety Costs

Looking closer at fatigue, we can peel away the layers to see that it includes some scary impairments, particularly when you consider that many fatigued people are flying our planes, trucking in our food, caring for us in hospitals, and policing our streets. These workers whose fatigue might be caused by chronic sleep deprivation, stress overload, and unhealthy lifestyles may be suffering from:

◆ Impaired alertness, communication skills, and judgment

◆ Decreased mental and physical performance

◆ Decreased vigilance and attentiveness

◆ Loss of logical reasoning skills and thinking ability

◆ Decreased or lost motor coordination

◆ Slowed reaction time

◆ General loss of awareness

Fatigued people, no matter what their role in life or their job, are just not as productive or safe due to the increase in human error fatigue causes. In fact, fatigue alone accounts for hundreds of billions of dollars every year due to accidents and increased medical-care costs.

Financial and Social Prices

Financial costs to employers aside, when you are fatigued it's not only difficult to perform at work, but you also might have more sick days or even periods of absence from work. In extreme cases, fatigue can cause you to be unable to continue working, resulting in loss of your livelihood.

Medical care in the United States isn't cheap, so when you add increased medical costs and decreased income, the result can be devastating. Some of the billions of dollars attributed to fatigue-related productivity loss also are coming out of your pocket.

When you turn down invitations from friends or cancel your appearance at social gatherings, life goes on and over time you can lose not only your job and your dreams, but your friends and social network.

Mind-Body Imbalance

Understanding the mind-body connection can help you to know how to maintain health and to see some of the reasons you become sick. It also can help you understand why Western medicine has a hard time with subjective symptoms and conditions such as fatigue. When you see a doctor, the focus is compartmentalized—sometimes only to one organ, depending on the doctor's specialty. But even in general or family practice, your doctor is looking for a specific condition to treat with medicine.

When people think of the mind-body connection, they often mistakenly believe that it relates only to how your emotions are affecting your health. Although this is true, the mind-body connection and mind-body balance is more accurately maintaining and supporting every aspect of your total being so you have *homeostasis* within every system.

def•i•ni•tion

Homeostasis refers to a system that is operated and maintained within its distinct and tolerable limits.

When one system goes out of whack, it affects other systems. So maintaining perfect health requires that each system is fed, fueled, oiled, rested, entertained, relaxed, massaged, filled with joy, and so on. If your heart or brain isn't happy, neither are other systems. No matter how well you are taking care of your body, if you are in emotional turmoil some system is going to become disrupted in order to try and clue you into addressing your emotional distress. To keep all your systems happy and functioning optimally, you not only have to feed and rest them properly, but you also can't stress them, overload them, or misuse them. It's a very fine-tuned balancing act that requires you giving each system the attention and care it requires.

Ever wonder what's up when you hear about the death of a long-distance runner? Aren't they supposed to be the epitome of heath? Well, consider that when a person is running 80 miles a week, some area most likely is neglected resulting in a mind-body imbalance. Overtraining doesn't allow for necessary rest and recuperation and often results in fatigue, which is a warning of potential injury. While the cause of death of long distance runners isn't usually cut and dry, and people who overtrain generally don't die from it, they can develop serious health problems.

In *Lore of Running*, author Tim Noakes, director of the University of Cape Town Medical Research Council Research Unit for Exercise Science & Sports Medicine, wrote, "Overtrained runners find that while their minds are ready to run, their bodies would much rather be asleep in bed. And the more their minds force them to train, the more their bodies resist until, in the race, the body has the final say." There is no getting around it. Every system in your body is entirely selfish and isn't going to compromise. They all insist on getting what they require, and when they don't, you pay, and fatigue is a common currency of mind-body imbalance.

In The Know

We still do not understand the cause of CFS, but studies around the world show that the illness involves real changes in the bodies of many patients. It is not "all in their heads."
—*Anthony Komaroff, M.D., Professor of Harvard Medical School*

Of course, good "mind" health, in the way of attitude and positive thinking, is absolutely essential for balance and homeostasis. But you cannot shoot yourself up with toxins and stressors while believing your life is a bowl of cherries and not get sick.

How Your Body Feels

Fatigue occurs on a continuum of severity from very mild to severe and crippling. Although the devastating fatigue of CFS is typically associated with a sudden onset, most people have mild fatigue that worsens as time goes by. We then classically turn to that always-handy denial to keep plowing through symptoms instead of dealing with them. So, when someone gets hit with the stressor that breaks the camel's back so to speak, that is what gets all the blame. The truth is that you are set up for the fall long before it happens.

Mild fatigue is something millions of people experience every day, and that may be why coffee is a multibillion dollar business. Severe fatigue, however, is absolutely incapacitating causing people to be bedridden and unable to do the most basic tasks, such as talking on the phone or brushing their teeth. This sort of debilitating fatigue is also known as *bone-crushing* fatigue because of its overwhelming nature.

Fatigue, over time, can get to the point that it is worsened by any physical or mental exertion or activity. And as fatigue worsens, so does the number and degree of other symptoms, including muscle and joint pain, nausea, diarrhea, gas, abdominal pain, sore throat, fever, chills, sweats, heat or cold intolerance, recurrent illness and infections, painful and/or swollen lymph nodes, and malaise (or that really crummy feeling you have when you are sick with the flu).

Weary, Worn-Out, and Drained

When fatigue is mild, it often feels somewhat like being tired, worn-out, or in a state of low energy. You feel like you are dragging and frequently wake up feeling run-down. It's tricky and deceiving because you don't feel in bad shape all the time, just off and on, and the amount of time that you feel yourself overshadows the low-energy times. It becomes second nature and you chock it up to getting older.

Mild fatigue becomes moderate fatigue. While you used to be dragging yourself through the day, you are now making excuses and bowing out of social events. You seem to have an affinity for the couch, you're not hitting the gym like you used to. But it's not because you don't want to, you tell yourself—you just need some time to relax. The amount of time that you feel worn-out is getting larger and the feel-good time is shrinking. You might start feeling worse after you push yourself to do things you enjoy. It's getting to be a head trip, so you begin to think it's not worth trying.

Moderate fatigue becomes severe fatigue when there is little or no amount of time when you feel well. You have days where you don't get out of bed at all. You still might be working, but you are freaked out that someone will find out that you are nearly comatose. The fact is that you are dangerous at work. You might be responsible for others' lives, you might be accountable for money, or you might even be in charge of your workplace or company.

You seriously question your abilities, with good cause, because you know that whatever it is that is wrong with you is having a serious impact. You can't explain it to anyone,

Slip-Ups

Stop thinking that your fatigue is due to your age because fatigue is never a healthy state at any age. It's noteworthy that people who care for their bodies and minds are not simply free-falling into old age. They don't have the mindset that age brings ill health.

and if you try, they just don't get it so you've stopped trying. You go to sleep thinking you will wake up feeling like yourself, but you wake up everyday feeling like someone shot you up with a heavy sedative. It might become too difficult to get up to take a shower or bath. You are seriously ill. Eventually, you can't kid yourself or anyone else, and you have to stop working. You are bedridden all of the time.

Muscle Weakness

The majority of people experience some degree of muscle weakness along with fatigue. Muscle weakness feels like a lack of strength and heaviness in the limbs. It refers to a lower capacity to exert force with your muscles like you should be able to given the state of your general physical fitness. More accurately, it's the physical component of fatigue.

When fatigue is mild, so is the muscle weakness. As fatigue progresses in severity, the muscles not only weaken, but also atrophy due to lack of use. Your muscles just don't operate like they should and, if you are severely fatigued, just lifting your arms over your head to shampoo your hair can feel like you are trying to lift a hundred pounds over your head.

Muscle fatigue varies from mild to profound. Muscles love to be exercised, and when you cannot they pay you back by becoming weak, which in turn leads to other problems including pain and increasing fatigue.

It Sometimes Hurts

It starts out with mild aches and pains that are easily ignored; your mom or grandpa had arthritis, remember? So you pop an occasional over-the-counter (OTC) pain reliever and get on with things. Time goes by and your fatigue starts getting worse, and so might your pain. Your muscles and joints ache, and your body is uncomfortable in weird places such as a sensation of burning, experiencing pressure beneath your breast bone, and experiencing chest pain. Then you begin to realize that you don't have any reason to ache the way you do and that resting or sleeping isn't helping. Your pain exhausts you further, it wears and tears at your ability to cope and to function, increasing your fatigue.

Pain does get worse over time, in part, due to a decrease in activity and because your muscles are beginning to atrophy. But you try to exercise and it seems only to make your fatigue worse, so you eventually give up and find yourself in that vicious circle of increased pain due to deconditioning and inability to exercise due to fatigue. What's a person to do?

Wired But Tired

An interesting but incredibly distressing phenomenon people with extreme fatigue experience is known as feeling "wired but tired." You are exhausted and, at times (if not all the time), in pain and anything you try to do requires Herculean effort. You cannot wait till night comes so you can get a good night's sleep and feel better in the morning. But when night comes, your body feels like a mass of concrete and twisted steel. You can't settle down. Your mind is racing. Your muscles are tense and may be burning, jumping, and twitching. You are, in fact, so tired that you can't think clearly. Too tired to do anything but lay there, too exhausted to read, but you are wide awake and end up tossing and turning.

As you lay there with your face and eyes twitching while breathing rapid and shallow breaths, you are overwhelmed with frustration, thinking "what is the deal?" The deal is that your homeostasis or internal balance is completely out of whack and at the same time you are not able to do enough during the day to actually truly physically and mentally tire yourself. You are without a doubt in a catch-22 situation. By the time you begin to experience wired but tired, it's hard to figure out if your insomnia caused your fatigue or if it was the other way around.

Energy Bar

To help deal with and prevent becoming wired but tired, plan on taking a relaxing walk in the evening followed by a soak in the tub. Avoid doing anything emotionally charged in the latter part of the day and evening, including animated conversations, dealing with bills, and watching TV.

Brain Fog

Fatigue doesn't just affect your muscles; it also affects your brain. Mental capacities are normally better when you are fresh and rested, and that's the thing about fatigue—you rarely if ever are. It's not that your skills at ripping out the *New York Times* crossword puzzle are worsening; it's that thinking is just getting harder and your short-term memory seems to be shot.

Depending on how fatigued you are, your ability to concentrate, multitask, or even remember where you parked your car may be compromised. That sharpest-knife-in-the-drawer mind of yours has turned into a dull, useless hatchet. And as your fatigue worsens, so does your cognitive (thinking) ability.

When you begin to lose your brain ability and you no longer associate your memory with a steel trap, you might begin to fear you have a brain tumor, Alzheimer's, or that you might have suffered a mild stroke or have some other mysterious neurological disease. Whatever is going on, you can't use denial like you did to ignore your tiredness and muscle weakness. This impairment isn't something you can ignore, it's your mind!

If you find yourself groping for words, frozen in time in front of your computer, not remembering what you were doing, or even forgetting whether you washed your hair while in the shower, you may be suffering from what is known as *brain fog*. Brain fog feels like you are thinking through cotton or dense fog. It's painful and hard sometimes to focus or concentrate. You're not drunk, but you feel loopy. It's getting harder to read and keep track of the plot. In fact, you seem to be losing the plot no matter how hard you try or what you are doing.

Brain function, when affected by fatigue, even can cause you to lose your balance and depth perception. You might have blurred vision and an increased sensitivity to light, sound, and odors. You may begin to feel that you are on overload and unable to deal with noise or groups of people, or are unable to understand directions when driving to a new place.

A huge number of people with severe fatigue experience brain fog. Of course, brain fog also can be caused by such things as the sometimes long-acting effects of general anesthesia and narcotic medications, anemia, numerous metabolic disorders, brain diseases, chemotherapy (chemo-brain), sleep disorders, hearing loss, stress, thyroid disease, psychiatric disorders, vitamin and other nutrient (omega-3 fatty acids) deficiencies, low blood sugar, food allergies, alcohol, and street drugs. And many of these factors in combination or independently also can be causing or aggravating your fatigue.

If you answer yes to all of the following questions, you definitely have brain fog. If you answer yes to some, you probably do. And if you cannot answer them at all, you have serious brain fog:

◆ Do you occasionally forget where you are?

◆ Do you find yourself saying a word that you didn't mean to say?

◆ When talking, do you sometimes lose the plot midsentence?

◆ Do the names of familiar objects frequently escape you?

◆ Are you frequently forgetting what you are doing, thinking, or talking about?

◆ Do the spellings of familiar words escape you?

◆ Is paperwork exhausting because you seem to be getting nowhere?

◆ Have your efficiency and organizational abilities gone down the drain?

It's important to note that any of the previous may be signs of early dementia (including Alzheimer's disease). So if you or any loved one is experiencing some increasing forgetfulness, an evaluation by a physician is in order.

How Does That Make You Feel?

You may be a type "A" personality, a high achiever, someone who burns the midnight oil, continually multitasks, runs marathons, and works a high-pressure job. And all of this can be slowly crumbling, or you might be dropping one thing at a time, not really understanding or having a reason why you cannot do the things that made you "YOU" for so many years. Fatigue can cause you to serious self-doubt while you are watching your identity slowly disappear. It's worth mentioning every way that fatigue is affecting you and your life when you see your doctor. This way your doctor can get a more accurate picture in order to help diagnose you.

Fatigue can take away your sense of control over your life and even your ability to dream and plan for the future. You feel helpless. You can't concentrate, and making decisions is difficult and sometimes downright impossible. You can't do some of the things you enjoy anymore because doing the things you need to do uses up any energy you have.

Slip-Ups

Just like your pill bottle instructs you, do not drive or operate heavy machinery while fatigued. Being fatigued carries the same dangers of being drunk.

Apathy, Moodiness, Irritability

Fatigue gets to be a serious head trip as time goes by, in part because it's such an effort to do anything. As things you once did with gusto are relegated to the wayside, you have mixed feelings of anger, worry, irritability, and apathy. You're worried about your inability to perform like you should, your friends just don't get it, people might be pressuring you about your responsibilities, and you feel angry and even a little scared. Because trying only causes you to crash and burn, you might even stop trying and throw in the towel.

Depression

Fatigue and lethargy are the most common and debilitating symptoms of depression, but what came first—the fatigue or depression? And are they in fact separate entities? Recent research has concluded that fatigue and lethargy are symptoms that continue even after symptoms of depression have disappeared. This might make you realize that, although depression may be one of those layers that needs to be addressed and peeled away, there are other causes of your fatigue that need a closer look as well.

Fatigue and depression mirror each other, and when you are experiencing one or both, it's hard to make a distinction because they both can be so incapacitating. Even though your fatigue might have come first, it's difficult to maintain good mental health when your life is so adversely affected.

If you were in a full-body cast, you would be getting a lot of support and caring from others. And although some might think a situation like that warrants support and attention more than that of fatigue, nothing is further from the truth. Fatigue is many times a frightening and incapacitating experience that comes at you seemingly without cause while stripping you of life as you know and desire it. Confusion, self-doubt, lack of support, validation, and understanding from others, and degree of disability from fatigue can in a susceptible person, lead to depression.

Anxiety and Worry

You can get by for a while sucking it up and not worrying about your performance, or bills for that matter. But you reach a point where you worry about everything because you are just not functioning. How will things get done, and what will the future hold since you have lost control? Whereas you used to worry about things that didn't matter, now you have serious cause to be concerned.

On top of real concerns, you also have issues related to your social life. What are you going to say for the tenth time to excuse yourself from a certain family or work function? Because fatigue isn't going away, you are feeling seriously roughed up and worries abound. Even though anxiety and worry can both contribute to fatigue and even depression, you can take back control over your life by decreasing the stressors that are causing your fatigue. As you continue to read on, remember that taking control means assuming personal responsibility over your health and doing what it takes to bring back balance to restore your energy and your health.

The Least You Need to Know

◆ Fatigue can be mild to severe and is a sense of weariness and tiredness that doesn't go away after a good night's sleep. Fatigue is not a healthy state but an indication that something (or many things) is amiss.

◆ Fatigue occurs in about one in four people at any given time—twice as often in women than men without any correlation to occupation or age.

◆ Fatigue causes impaired alertness, communication skills, and judgment; decreased mental and physical performance; decreased vigilance and attentiveness; a loss of logical reasoning skills and thinking ability; decreased or lost motor coordination; slowed reaction time; and general loss of awareness.

◆ Mind-body balance and connection is about maintaining and supporting, while not stressing, misusing, or overburdening, every aspect of your total being so that you have homeostasis (perfect balance) within every system. Emotions can affect physical health and vice versa.

◆ As fatigue worsens, so does the number and degree of other symptoms, including muscle and joint paint, nausea, diarrhea, gas, abdominal pain, sore throat, fever, chills, sweats, heat or cold intolerance, recurrent illness and infections, painful and/or swollen lymph nodes, and malaise (that really crummy feeling you have when you are sick with the flu).

◆ Fatigue may cause or worsen insomnia and depression and may be accompanied by cognitive symptoms such as brain fog.

Chapter 2

Physiological Causes

In This Chapter

- ◆ Unraveling physical causes
- ◆ How illness and infection fit in
- ◆ Understanding the toxic soup we live in
- ◆ Getting to the bottom of your lack of sleep

The cause of your fatigue may be multilayered, but at the bottom of it all, you have to look at any possible physical causes. By first addressing and treating any illness or condition you might be dealing with, you will then have the energy to deal with some of the other factors that are getting you down. A number of potential factors can be contributing to the physical causes of your fatigue, and this chapter covers several them. Taking a look at the conditions discussed in this chapter should give you some clues as to what you need to include in your final plan of action and some of the steps you need to take to win your fight.

Low Blood Sugar (Hypoglycemia)

Hypoglycemia is not a disease; it's a constellation of symptoms that indicate low blood sugar. This syndrome is more accurately described as the body's inability to properly handle sugar causing symptoms that may include fatigue, irritability, nervousness, depression, insomnia, flushing, impaired memory and concentration, anxiety, sweating, headache, dizziness, faintness or fainting, and more.

The best treatment for those suffering from hypoglycemia is to adhere to a diet that steers clear of certain carbohydrate foods that are high in refined or simple carbs. There is more information on this in Chapter 11.

Infections

Infections caused by yeast, bacteria, parasites, or viruses can also cause fatigue. If your infection goes unnoticed or untreated, as chronic infections sometimes do, your fatigue may come on gradually and you may not associate it with any infection. Or if you recover from an infection, you might have a post-infectious syndrome that causes what is referred to as a *hit-and-run injury* to your brain and immune system.

Energy Bar _____

Researchers believe that causative factors such as infections (and allergies and stress) possibly could deplete the body's stores of adenosine triphosphate (ATP) that's necessary to supply energy to cells, resulting in fatigue. For this reason, some people with fatigue improve when they take a nicotinamide adenine dinucleotide (NADH) supplement. NADH is a coenzyme in cells that helps in the process of energy production.

Many people with chronic fatigue also have elevated levels of antibodies indicating exposure to or past infection of Lyme disease, candida (or yeast infection), Herpes virus type 6, human T-cell lymphotropic virus, Epstein-Barr virus, measles, coxsackie B, cytomegalovirus, or parvovirus. But so far, no one infectious agent has been identified to cause Chronic Fatigue Syndrome (CFS) or post-infectious syndrome; however, a majority of cases of CFS do begin with a flulike illness.

It's now known that some people with CFS have a chronic enteroviral infection that causes persistent or intermittent upper and or lower gastrointestinal symptoms. Enterovirus infection is associated with CFS but is still thought to be actually caused by other factors, including a previous or ongoing viral infection, compromised immune function, and the cumulative effects of fatigue stressors over time. Fatigue stressors, which we look at more closely in Chapter 14, include a poor diet; dysfunctional relationships; inadequate sleep, rest, or nutrients; excessive behaviors; medical conditions including addictions; overuse of medications; toxic lifestyle habits and choices; and environmental toxins.

Post-infectious syndrome is a period of prolonged fatigue related to a prior viral illness such as infectious mononucleosis. For most people post-infectious syndrome becomes a low-level feeling of being run-down or fatigued, but for others it can result in the devastating fatigue of CFS. Where exactly a person is located on the continuum of fatigue, from mild to severe, directly correlates with his level of immune function. Factors that weaken immune function are the fatigue stressors that we look at all through this book: poor diet and lifestyle habits, lack of sufficient rest, excessive and unhealthy behaviors, and toxins that poison and tax the body.

Leaky Gut Syndrome

Some researchers believe that mercury toxicity from such things as a high level of mercury in the diet or dental amalgams are associated with chronic infection of the GI tract (gut). The stress of this or any other toxicity, including overuse of over-the-counter (OTC) and prescription medications and antibiotics, along with the typical Standard American Diet (SAD), often causes what is known as leaky gut syndrome.

According to the American Dental Association (ADA), silver fillings are safe. However, the ADA, the Environmental Protection Agency (EPA), and the Occupational Safety and Health Administration (OSHA) have very rigid guidelines for the handling and disposal of mercury after it is removed from your mouth. These agencies all consider your old fillings to be toxic waste! Because the controversy has never really been settled, it's up to you to make a personal choice in regard to using this material in your mouth.

Although not an established medical diagnosis in conventional medicine, leaky gut syndrome is thought by some researchers to arise when the lining of the GI tract becomes compromised and develops microscopic holes that allow bacteria, toxins, and foreign particles to leak into the body. They are then recognized as foreign invaders and further tax the immune system.

A leaky gut causes fatigue and bloating because it doesn't properly absorb nutrients and foods. The body is flooded continually with foreign proteins crossing the leaky membrane, so a person also can develop food allergies, chemical sensitivity, nutritional deficiencies, infections, and autoimmune diseases.

Allergies

Allergies are a common affliction affecting about one out of every three people. An allergic reaction is an acquired abnormal inflammatory reaction to a substance (allergen) caused by environmental agents. Common allergens include dust, dust mites, pollen, mold, pet dander, cockroaches, insect stings and bites, medications, certain foods, and personal care and household products.

def•i•ni•tion

Anaphylaxis is a sudden severe, whole-body allergic reaction that is life-threatening. It can occur in response to any allergen. **Sensitization** is the process where over time a person becomes increasingly allergic to an allergen as a result of repeated exposure.

Allergies are common in all age groups, and allergic reactions range in severity from mild to a life-threatening allergic reaction called *anaphylaxis*. Even though a person might not have experienced any reaction or only very mild reactions to an allergen for many years, sometimes repeated exposures, or *sensitization*, eventually leads to a more severe reaction without any warning.

Allergies arise when your body's defensive system, the immune system, comes into contact with something it interprets as a foreign substance and a threat. Sometimes the immune system works to protect your body, but other times it has difficulty distinguishing between actual threats and substances that are not threats. Those hyperreactive systems tend to react with an inflammatory response to substances that aren't actually harmful, such as certain foods. Dairy, corn, eggs, citrus, and food additives are common sources of food allergies. And these days, due to the continual barrage of chemicals, many people who would not normally have allergy problems do now because their immune systems are in overdrive from the continual onslaught of toxins.

Allergies manifest with various symptoms, including skin and respiratory problems, hives, sinusitis, hay fever, and asthma. They also are a well-known cause of fatigue and mental symptoms including mood changes, memory and concentration problems, sleep disturbances, depression, and anxiety. Allergic reactions can cause an overall feeling of malaise because, in essence, the reaction is "sickness" and energy depleting because your immune system is continually fighting what is seen as a foreign invader. And allergies often also affect your sleep, causing you to become chronically fatigued.

Pollution

It is all around us in the air we breath. Sometimes you can see it; sometimes you can't. But it is almost impossible to avoid. Although it is commonplace in large cities, the countryside is not immune to its existence. It's air pollution.

It is something you would expect to see if you traveled to Los Angeles or Mexico City, but this abnormal, visible or invisible substance can be found anywhere and is a threat to the health of human beings, other life, and the earth itself.

In The Know
"Smog is a soup that contains a lot of stuff, and people inhale everything that's in it, a whole bunch of toxic chemicals, they're a significant threat to people's health." —Daniel Menzel, M.D., Ph.D., professor in the Department of Community and Environmental Medicine at the University of California, Irvine.

The primary components of air pollution consist of ozone, carbon monoxide, nitrous oxides, particulate matter, sulfur dioxide, and lead. These pollutants come from sources such as coal-burning power plants and industries, refineries, power plants burning fossil fuels, diesel engines, motor vehicles, dust, and wood- and coal-burning stoves.

Breathing smog causes the lungs to become hypersensitive, reacting with inflammation, bronchial spasms, coughing, asthma attacks, and increased mucus production. Smog decreases your immune function by making lung cells vulnerable to attack from bacteria and viruses present in the air and causes eye, lung, and respiratory problems. The general malaise and fatigue many people feel with symptoms including headaches, dizziness, and shortness of breath can be due, in part, from breathing contaminated air.

Chemical Sensitivity

Multiple chemical sensitivity (MCS) has not yet been proven to be a valid medical condition. However, there are more reports from sufferers as time goes on describing it as an overwhelming, continual state of acute sensitivity or allergic response that typically begins after either an acute or a chronic exposure to toxic chemicals. Symptoms of MCS are many and varied and include fatigue, headaches, flulike symptoms, nausea and other GI problems, breathing problems, muscle and joint pain, dry and burning eyes, rashes, and cognitive difficulties.

It's thought MCS has emerged due to the increased use of *volatile organic compounds (VOCs)*. The level of VOCs is almost always higher indoors than outdoors due to the use of pesticides; perfumes and other fragrant products; fuels; carpets; building materials; paints; lacquers; paint strippers; office supplies, equipment, and materials; cleaning supplies; and furnishings. VOCs also are emitted by new cars and are essentially what make up that "new car smell."

def•i•ni•tion

Volatile organic compounds (VOCs) are toxic chemicals capable of escaping and saturating the air as a sort of chemical gas. Because toxins are fat-soluble, those that compose VOCs enter the body through the lungs, eyes, mucous membranes, and skin and saturate the lipid tissues of the body, including the brain and cell membranes that are largely composed of fat.

The adverse health effects of VOCs vary from highly toxic and carcinogenic to minimal health effects depending on the level of exposure and length of time exposed. Some VOCs are suspected and some are known causes of cancer. Many people who have continual symptoms like unexplained headaches or low-level, allergy-type symptoms and fatigue are really experiencing the adverse effects of exposure to VOCs.

Because of the continual bombardment of VOCs, a singe assault such as contact with new carpeting, a carpet cleaning, or a flea bombing of your house can be enough to kick off MCS.

Household and Personal Care Products

Household and personal care products are another reason for unexplained MSC, fatigue, chronic headaches, allergies, sinus problems, joint pain, chronic breathing difficulties, dizziness, numbness and tingling, inability to concentrate, pain, frequent infections, or any other vague symptom your doctor is unable to diagnose. Everywhere you go, from the workplace to shopping to school, you are barraged with chemical and biological pollutants that add to your toxic load and decreased quality of life.

No one is immune to the cumulative toxic effects of chemicals, including those that make up fragrances in household cleaners as well as in personal care products like shampoo, hair spray, and perfume. Toxic chemicals enter the body by inhalation; absorption through the skin, eyes, and mucous membranes; and ingestion.

Products that say they are safe do not consider the fact that you are using hundreds of other products. Because so many chemicals are used in so many products, you can experience a cumulative effect of exposures to multiple products over time. Houses, clothing, and bodies that have an overlying smell created from chemicals used to clean or create or mask odors are creating a chemical soup in your body. Consider the use of dryer sheets—not only are you emitting VOCs into your home and the atmosphere, but when you wear that clothing with its thin layer of chemicals next to your skin, you are also allowing those toxins to be absorbed while you inhale the VOCs it emits.

The active ingredient in personal care products and antimicrobial soaps—methylisothiazolinone—is known to cause nerve damage that may be adding to the epidemic of learning disorders and hyperactivity in children and Alzheimer's disease in adults. And you can't ever really protect yourself from the nonsterile, microorganism-laden environment you live in by washing with chemical-laden soaps that also wash away your protective flora. What keeps you healthy is an immune system that is supported by the right nutrition and that is not taxed by stressors like toxins.

Other substances found in products are chemicals known as endocrine disruptors, which disrupt natural body hormones by acting like hormones found in the endocrine system. The endocrine system is a sophisticated and intricate system that controls maturation, development, growth, and regulation within the body by synthesizing hormones, the body's natural chemical messengers.

Slip-Ups

Don't believe that that scented plug-in, candle, or air freshener will bring you peace and tranquility because the VOCs it emits will most likely only give you a headache, nasal stuffiness, and fatigue.

Endocrine disruptors present in synthetic materials, such as pesticides, plastics, body creams, detergents, and food supplies, fool the body into processing them as if they were estrogens, interrupting or interfering with this finely regulated hormonal messenger system. These compounds mimic natural hormones and can cause reproductive or developmental problems. Some researchers believe these hormone masqueraders are adding to the current epidemic of chronic illness.

Most endocrine disruptor chemicals are fat-soluble and, after they enter the body, they are stored in fat. Researchers today agree that there is a potential of possible damage to health from exposure to endocrine disruptors and are stepping up research efforts. The evidence of harm has come from adverse effects seen in wildlife and laboratory animals, along with worrying changes in certain health trends in humans.

In The Know

"Humankind is facing a pandemic of endocrine-related disorders that can seriously alter the quality of life, and the world economy and stability. Scientists have demonstrated that some synthetic chemicals can cause the same disorders that have rapidly become major public health concerns."

—*Theo Colborn, Ph.D., coauthor of* Our Stolen Future: Are We Threatening Our Fertility, Intelligence, and Survival? A Scientific Detective Story.

Obesity

Obesity is a well-known risk factor for many health conditions and the cause of symptoms including fatigue and decreased quality of life. According to the National Institutes of Health (NIH), a person is obese with a *body mass index (BMI)* of 30 and above—typically 30 or more pounds overweight.

Obesity is a complicated problem that robs people of their energy, further compounding their ability to be active. Someone carrying around 70 extra pounds is going to have a lot more wear and tear on her joints and will most likely tire faster than someone of normal weight. People often throw in the towel on doing normal activities because it's just too tiring. They then may self-medicate with their drug of choice (food), and the vicious cycle is maintained.

def•i•ni•tion

Body Mass Index (BMI) is a reliable numerical indicator of body fat that is calculated from a person's weight and height. Knowing your BMI is a good way to watch weight factors that may lead to health problems. See Appendix C for Internet sites where you can calculate your BMI.

While some people have genetic differences in their fat storage cells causing excessive fat storage, others are obese simply due to overeating. People who overeat typically consume too many calories of unhealthy foods along with sedentary lifestyles that together result in obesity.

Of course, there are many reasons people overeat, but a diet of junk and processed foods is a major perpetuating factor for obesity. These foods typically are loaded with calories and the additives in processed foods not only increase the craving for food, but also do not signal satiety in the body like real, whole food does.

Obesity goes hand in hand with other perpetuating problems for fatigue including sleep apnea, other sleep disorders, and chronic pain.

Male and Female Menopause

While female menopause issues have always been hot topics, male menopause is just beginning to arise as a valid concern. When men go through male menopause, or *andropause*, their testosterone levels begin to drop; thus, by age 60 their testosterone levels are only a fraction of what they were in early adulthood. As the testosterone level gradually begins to drop beginning around age 30, changes gradually occur, such as loss of muscle mass and virility, decreased energy, and increased fatigue.

Women go through a natural stage of life called *menopause* when their ovaries stop producing eggs, causing estrogen and progesterone levels to change and menstruation to end. Menopause technically occurs when it has been one year since a woman's final menstrual period, typically around age 51. Female menopause occurs during a period in midlife and causes physical changes and emotional symptoms such as fatigue, hot spells, sweating, sadness, depression, and many other symptoms.

Managing menopause for both sexes is covered in Chapter 13.

Sleep Disorders

You know how important getting a good night's rest is for feeling good in the morning. If you wake up fatigued, you might be suffering from a sleep disorder.

Sleep disorders (covered more thoroughly in Chapter 12) interfere with your ability to get your required sleep. It might be hard for you to fall asleep or stay asleep all through the night. You may wake up feeling tired or feel sleepy during the day even though you feel you got enough sleep.

Although there are more than 80 known sleep disorders, some of the most common sleep disorders are insomnia, sleep apnea, and Restless Legs Syndrome.

Insomnia

Every night, millions of people lay awake counting sheep unable to fall asleep. Some people fall asleep without any problem but don't stay asleep, and others simply toss and turn. None of these people get a "good night's sleep" due to what is commonly known as *insomnia* or *disorders of initiating and maintaining sleep (DIMS)*.

Someone suffering from insomnia has difficulty falling and staying asleep. To make things worse, once asleep, their quality of sleep often is poor, despite having adequate sleeping time. This is classified as a sleep disorder when it's also accompanied by day-time sleepiness, anxiety about sleep, loss of concentration, irritability, loss of motivation, or any other daytime impairment that can be associated with the sleep problem.

Insomnia can be transient (lasting a week or less), short-term (lasting one to six months), or chronic (lasting six months or longer). It's the most common sleep disorder and affects 10 to 15 percent of Americans.

This struggle to sleep usually is caused by a mishmash of factors including the use of alcohol and drugs, psychological and physical predisposition, bad habits, uncomfortable environments, and negative conditioning.

People who are physically predisposed to insomnia might have a hyperactive arousal system. Their brains are supersensitive, their hearts beat faster, their body temperature is higher, and any sort of noise or disturbance can startle them awake. Those with a psychological predisposition might be more anxious and easily stressed and, because they don't react well to stress or problems, a little insomnia can send them into a tailspin of worry.

Although used by millions, any drug (including sleeping pills and alcohol) only works to disrupt sleep. These drugs cause shorter, more disturbed sleeping patterns and inhibit the production of dopamine, the brain's neurotransmitter that promotes sleep. Self-medicating causes a revolving door of worsening insomnia and increased drug and alcohol use in an attempt to compensate, which often leaves a person both sleep deprived and addicted. Some tranquilizers and sleep-inducing drugs *are* beneficial for insomnia, but they need to be prescribed by a doctor and accompany a good treatment plan that includes changing sleep habits, good sleep hygiene, and an understanding of the drug's use.

Sleep Apnea

There are two types of sleep apnea: central and obstructive, with the latter being the most common. Obstructive sleep apnea (OSA) occurs when the upper airways collapse while asleep and obstruct the flow of air; after continual efforts to breathe, the breathing stops for a period of seconds to a minute or more. Then after a loud snort or choking sound, breathing begins again. These brief breathing pauses occur over and over during the night and are often accompanied by a drop in oxygen levels in the blood; deep sleep is interrupted and poor sleep quality results. Those with central sleep apnea (CSA) have the same symptoms of breathing cessation, but it's caused by a lack of appropriate signals from the brain to the breathing muscles for respiration.

Without treatment, people with sleep apnea can develop high blood pressure, cardio-vascular disease, memory problems, weight gain, impotency, and headaches. Untreated sleep apnea can be responsible for daytime impairment from ongoing fatigue that causes poor job performance, accidents, and decreased quality of life.

Restless Legs Syndrome

Restless Legs Syndrome (RLS) is a neurological disorder. Those who suffer from RLS have sensations in the legs that cause uncontrollable urges to move in an attempt to relieve, minimize, or prevent the unpleasant feelings. These sensations can be uncomfortable, irritating, and even painful and feel like creeping, tugging, burning, or insects crawling under the skin.

These sensations typically happen when lying down to relax or sleep, causing the person difficulty falling and staying asleep. This can result in exhaustion and fatigue that typically affects work performance, relationships, and quality of life. RLS affects all ages but occurs most frequently in the middle-aged or older persons. The severity of symptoms increases with age. RLS is often accompanied by periodic limb movement disorder (PLMD), or the repetitive and uncontrollable cramping or jerking of the legs while asleep that causes frequent awakening and disrupted sleep.

For some, RLS symptoms are less evident during the day and increase in severity in the evening or at night. Sometimes the symptoms dissipate by early morning so the person is able to then get more refreshing sleep. Periods of inactivity that can trigger the symptoms include long car trips, sitting for long periods, air travel, relaxation exercises, or a period of immobilization due to having a limb in a cast.

RLS can result in restlessness, the inability to sit still, difficulty falling asleep and/or staying asleep, daytime impairment, and chronic fatigue.

Hypothyroid

You might be one of the millions of people who are fatigued, experiencing hair loss, gaining weight, and depressed but don't feel you should mention these symptoms to your doctor because you attribute them to age, lack of exercise, and poor lifestyle habits.

Some of the many symptoms of hypothyroid are fatigue and weakness; low temperature or cold intolerance; dry, coarse skin; hair loss; cold hands and feet; weight gain; insomnia; constipation; depression; memory problems; dementia; nervousness; tremors; problems with your immune system; and heavy menstrual periods.

def•i•ni•tion

The **thyroid** gland produces and stores hormones that work to regulate the heart rate, blood pressure, body temperature, and metabolism. These hormones are essential for the overall functioning of the body.

Several factors can put you at risk for *thyroid* disease. You are at a higher risk if you have a family member with a thyroid problem; you currently have a pituitary, endocrine, or autoimmune disease (or have these diseases in your family); you have CFS or Fibromyalgia; you are female; you are over 60 years of age; you have just had a baby; you are near or in menopause; you smoke; you've had radiation exposure; you've been treated with lithium; or you've been exposed to certain chemicals.

Although thyroid disease is common, some believe it's even more prevalent than numbers show despite the newer guidelines. It's often still underdiagnosed, patients are often misunderstood, and the condition often goes untreated.

Anemia

Anemia is one of the more common blood disorders that occurs when the number of red blood cells (RBCs) is below normal. RBCs contain hemoglobin, and their job is to carry oxygen to the cells. Less hemoglobin results in lower oxygen levels in cells, leading to fatigue and then to other health problems.

You may or may not have any symptoms with mild anemia, or if you do have symptoms, you might be attributing them to other things. The signs of mild anemia can be subtle but can include the following:

◆ Chronic fatigue or irritability

◆ Frequent headaches

◆ Loss of appetite

◆ Constipation that occurs without any changes in eating habits

◆ A very pale skin color, or if you have a dark skin your lips might be pale or your skin look "washed out"

◆ Difficulty concentrating, which might be affecting your ability to function at work or school

◆ A craving for unusual foods (pica), including eating strange nonfoods like soil, clay, and paper

◆ Depression

◆ Shortness of breath

◆ Feelings of coldness in the extremities

◆ Weakness and/or dizziness

There are many causes of anemia, but the most common is iron deficiency. If you have any suspicions that you may be anemic, you need to see your doctor for a routine blood test, most commonly a hemoglobin (the protein in red blood cells that carries oxygen) or a hematocrit (the number and the size of red blood cells) or both. Don't wait until you develop signs such as a sore tongue, sores in your mouth, or a stoppage in your menstrual cycle because by then your anemia will have become long-standing. Severe anemia has significant health consequences particularly affecting the heart.

Slip-Ups

Most people are familiar with iron deficiency anemia. You need iron to make hemoglobin. Iron deficiency anemia must be diagnosed and treated by a doctor. Never take iron supplements except under a doctor's supervision because iron overloading can be dangerous and cause damage to your liver among other adverse health consequences.

Anemia is not a disease but a symptom of many diseases. Some of these diseases (but not all) are dietary. Once anemia (low red cell levels) is determined, then a number of tests may need to be done to figure out the root cause. If you are anemic, to properly treat you your doctor will need to determine the source by testing your blood. Be sure to tell your doctor all the signs and symptoms you are experiencing and, in the meantime, begin to focus on any dietary changes that might be causing your symptoms. See Chapter 10 for ways the you can use diet and nutrition as a means to stay healthy.

The Least You Need to Know

◆ Hypoglycemia is an inability to properly handle sugar that causes symptoms of fatigue, irritability, nervousness, depression, insomnia, flushing, impaired memory and concentration, anxiety, sweating, headache, dizziness, faintness or fainting, and many other symptoms.

◆ Chronic infections and infections you've recovered from but that cause a hit-and-run injury to your brain and immune system are both causes of fatigue.

◆ Air pollution, environmental toxics, chemicals in products, and allergies are causes of fatigue in many people.

◆ Obesity is a well-known risk factor for many health conditions and causes symptoms that include fatigue and decreased quality of life.

◆ Both men and women experience menopause at different times with different physiological causes, but both can result in symptoms of loss of energy and fatigue.

◆ Anemia and hypothyroidism are two common treatable conditions with symptoms of fatigue.

Chapter 3

Serious Fatigue Diseases

In This Chapter

◆ Looking at some fatiguing illnesses more closely

◆ Fatigue goes hand in hand with some treatments

◆ A glimpse of certain posttreatment effects

◆ Fatigue might be due to your medication

Cancer and multiple sclerosis are considered accepted diagnosis by the medical community. However, some of the other fatiguing illnesses such as adrenal fatigue and Chronic Fatigue Syndrome (CFS) that, though devastating, have not been accepted diagnoses by some medical care providers. In addition to a lack of validation and support by their medical team, some people, despite being very sick, also lack support from their friends and families. This is due in part to the lack of credibility that comes from the dismissal of these conditions from the medical team and because there has not been enough media attention and awareness efforts focused on some of these very real (and in some cases devastating) illnesses.

There is mounting evidence that some of the more invisible illnesses that cannot be proved by lab tests do indeed exist and are in fact supported by such agencies as the Center for Disease Control (CDC) and by Medicare. This chapter briefly outlines some of the common, serious fatigue-related diseases; gives you some validation of some of your symptoms; and provides information as to how this information relates to your fatigue.

You might have been diagnosed with a serious condition that causes fatigue and, if you have a serious disease, you have to work even harder to conquer symptoms like fatigue. If you apply all the measures outlined in this book to address what I call fatigue stressors, such as improving a poor diet and eliminating toxins in what you eat and in your environment, you can still win some battles and improve your fatigue even if you don't win the war.

There is no known medical cure for CFS. Most doctors will only offer treatment aimed at symptom relief and improving day-to-day functioning. Although CFS is known by experts to be as crippling as end-stage AIDS or as debilitating as cancer chemotherapy, people who developed CFS prior to recent times have had to endure years of emotional trauma in addition to their physical suffering because of not having the validation and support of their doctors and even friends and family.

These days, if your doctor doesn't support you, there are many others who will. So be sure to seek one of them out. The best CFS treatments are the measures that are outlined throughout this book, along with the support of your family doctor and your loved ones and friends. Because documentation regarding CFS has been vague, the recovery from it is also unknown. However, many experts agree that you can recover within two years after your symptoms begin improving.

Multiple Sclerosis

Multiple sclerosis (MS) is an *autoimmune disease* of the central nervous system (CNS) that ranges from very mild with little or no symptoms to having some disabling features to devastating.

def•i•ni•tion

In **autoimmune diseases,** your immune system mounts an attack against your own tissues causing inflammation and damage resulting in autoimmune disorders. These autoimmune disorders can affect connective tissue, nerves, muscles, and the endocrine and digestive systems.

In MS, the body mistakenly attacks the proteins in the fatty substance (myelin sheath) that insulate the nerve fibers of the brain and spinal cord, causing inflammation and injury to the sheath and eventually the nerves. The resulting scar tissue (sclerosis) interferes with the nerve's ability to transmit electrical impulses back and forth between the brain and the body.

The majority of people with MS experience their first symptom between the ages of 20 and 40. Typically, blurred or double vision, red-green color distortion, or blindness in one eye is the initial cause for concern. Other symptoms include muscle weakness in the extremities, difficulty with coordination and balance, transitory numbness, or pins and needles sensations. Some people experience pain, speech impediments, tremors, dizziness, and paralysis. The variety of symptoms depends on the area of the body where the nerve communication is damaged.

Fatigue, both mental and physical, is believed to be the most common symptom of MS and seemingly unrelated to the level of disability. Mental fatigue tends to be worsened by exercise or increased body or environmental temperature.

Physical fatigue can be caused by something like a short walk or any other physical activity. The ability to function can decrease with activity, so when the person tries to go for a walk for example, he might start out feeling fine and then end up not being able to lift his foot to take a step. Pushing beyond the person's limits, whatever they may be, seriously exhausts or disables him further and his recovery times will vary depending on the level of the disability.

There is as yet no cure for MS, but various medications are used for treatment, although some people choose to not have therapy due to the risk of medication side effects. Overall, though, some tend to do well.

Cancer

Tumors occur when cells grow when they shouldn't or old cells that should die don't and these two abnormal processes form a mass that is known as a *tumor*. Tumors can be *benign* (not cancer) or *malignant* (cancer). Some tumors stay put where they originated, and some spread to other areas of the body—called *metastasis*. Symptoms of cancer depend on the cancer type and the stage, or how advanced it is, and the treatments include surgery, radiation, and chemotherapy. For the more than 100 types of cancer, each has its own symptoms, characteristics, and effect on the body. Fatigue, however, is one of the most commonly experienced symptoms of both the disease and the treatments.

According to the American Cancer Society, one million cancer diagnoses occur every year, with one out of two men and one out of three women having a cancer diagnosis in their lifetime. Although cancer can occur at any age and in any race or ethnic group, the majority occurs in people age 55 and older.

Even though millions of people have beat cancer or are living with it, the best approach to avoiding an encounter with cancer is to adopt the fatigue stressor elimination measures that are outlined in Part 3 of this book. Healthy lifestyle choices such as getting enough sleep, removing toxins and supporting your immune and other body systems with the proper nutrition, and pleasure in life are not only healing, but are preventative measures for all adverse health conditions.

Hepatitis B and C

Hepatitis B is a *chronic* (long-term) or *acute* (short-term) liver infection that is caused by the hepatitis B virus. The hepatitis B virus is transmitted through infected blood or other body fluids from people who have hepatitis B (HBV). You can get HBV by having unprotected sex with an infected person or by sharing needles with someone who has the virus, or if you are health-care worker and accidentally get stuck with a needle that was used on an infected patient. Infected women also can pass the virus on to their babies when they are pregnant. You can't get HBV from shaking hands or hugging an infected person.

Symptoms of hepatitis B range from mild to severe and include fatigue, nausea, vomiting, loss of appetite, abdominal pain, jaundice (yellow skin), weakness, and brown colored urine.

Acute hepatitis lasts six weeks or less, but in some people it becomes a chronic illness. This typically occurs in 10 to 20 percent of people who are infected and have a liver that has been damaged from the acute illness, making it unable to recover. Some people with chronic HBV have no symptoms, although it can still lead to cirrhosis (scarring and fatty deposits) of the liver. People with cirrhosis can't cleanse their bodies of wastes, and cirrhosis can progress to liver failure and even liver cancer.

HBV is diagnosed with blood tests; in some cases, a liver biopsy also might be needed. Avoiding unprotected sex and not sharing needles is the best way to prevent HBV infection. In addition, a vaccine is available to prevent HBV. If you have chronic HBV, you might choose to undergo available treatments and, depending on the severity of your infection and treatment response, the treatment can take a year or more.

Energy Bar

If you have HBV or HCV, you can live a healthier life with either disease and improve your chances of clearing the virus with treatment by addressing the fatigue stressors in your life, giving your liver and immune system their best shot.

Hepatitis C (HCV) is a viral infection of the liver that can lead to serious permanent liver damage (cirrhosis), liver failure, liver cancer, and even death. HCV was first identified in 1989 and, unlike other viral hepatitis, it is more difficult for the immune system to overcome. Thus, 85 percent or more of infected persons develop a chronic infection. The time from infection to the development of serious liver damage can take 20 years or longer. HCV is transmitted from only infected blood to blood, and prior to 1990 before blood was adequately tested, blood transfusions accounted for nearly 10 percent of all cases.

Transmission of the HCV occurs with IV drug use, poorly sterilized medical instruments, blood spills, tattooing or body piercing, shared razors or toothbrushes, body fluids like mucous that contain infected blood, and needle sticks. However, no risk factors are evident in about 10 percent of the cases. Note that even if a tattoo is done with a sterilized needle, the ink that was used might have been contaminated! In a small percent of cases, infected women can transmit the virus to their unborn babies.

The symptoms of HCV are sometimes mild or nonexistent, but the most common symptom is fatigue. Other symptoms include mild fever, muscle and joint pain, nausea, vomiting, loss of appetite, indistinct abdominal pain, and sometimes diarrhea. Some people remain undiagnosed because their symptoms feel like a flu bug that comes and goes or because they never develop any symptoms at all. But even without symptoms, a person with chronic HCV can develop liver damage.

Because HCV is a relatively new disease, there are many people who have experienced symptoms such as profound fatigue that have interfered drastically with their lives, but this fatigue wasn't validated by their medical team. It's just in recent years that researchers have come to find that fatigue is the most common and sometimes disabling symptom of HCV, regardless of whether a person has liver damage.

There is no vaccine for HCV, and because the virus mutates, it might be a very long time before one is available. HCV can be diagnosed using a blood test, or a liver biopsy in some cases. Depending on factors including length of infection, age, disease progression, and other variables, people might opt to undergo treatment. Treatment is generally 24 or 48 weeks in duration, depending on the "strain" or genotype of HCV virus the person has. Some people have extended treatments beyond the standard times due to other factors. Because HCV progresses slowly, many people can live a long life with chronic HCV; other people can even undergo successful treatment, clear the virus, and recover completely.

The CDC estimates that more than one million Americans are chronically infected with HBV and three to four million Americans are chronically infected with HCV. HCV is the leading cause of cirrhosis and liver failure, and the main reason for liver transplants in the United States. And because you can live for decades with no symptoms, it's recommended that you be tested if you have had any risk factors for infection in your lifetime.

Chronic Fatigue Syndrome

According to the CDC, CFS affects more than one million Americans and there are millions of people who, although they don't fully meet the strict research criteria for CFS, have equally incapacitating fatiguing illnesses. CFS is a complex and debilitating illness that is primarily characterized by profound fatigue that doesn't improve with rest or sleep and is typically worsened by physical or mental activity (post exertional fatigue) that lasts more than 24 hours.

Persons with CFS also have other symptoms including brain fog, weakness, a feeling of high body temperature, pain, alcohol intolerance, night sweats, depression, irritability, anxiety and panic attacks, shortness of breath, abnormal skin sensations, tingling sensations, weight loss, and many other symptoms.

def•i•ni•tion

The Epstein-Barr virus (EBV) causes **mononucleosis,** also known as "mono" or the "kissing disease." Although EBV can be associated in some cases, it does not cause CFS. CFS is a separate disorder and is not merely EBV infection or long-term mononucleosis.

CFS feels like a chronic bad flu or *mononucleosis*. It's sometimes associated with infections, but so far there isn't any proof that it's caused by a virus or other infectious organism. People with CFS can be sick for years; causes have not been identified, and there are no specific diagnostic tests. Your doctor will diagnosis you with CFS usually only when all the other conditions that can cause fatigue are ruled out and you meet the criteria for diagnosis as laid out by the CDC.

To be diagnosed with CFS, you must have severe chronic fatigue for six months or longer with other medical conditions and have four or more of the following symptoms:

◆ Significant impairment in short-term memory or concentration

◆ Sore throat

◆ Tender lymph nodes

◆ Muscle pain and/or multijoint pain without swelling or redness

◆ Headaches of a new type, pattern, or severity

◆ Unrefreshing sleep

◆ Post exertional malaise (fatigue or feeling sick or flulike) that lasts more than 24 hours

Some researchers insist that CFS can be diagnosed only if the following conditions are excluded:

◆ Sleep apnea and narcolepsy

◆ Chronic mononucleosis

◆ Hypothyroidism

◆ Major depressive disorders

◆ Bipolar affective disorders

◆ Schizophrenia

◆ Eating disorders

◆ Cancer

◆ Autoimmune disease

◆ Some hormonal disorders

◆ Subacute infections

◆ Obesity

◆ Alcohol or substance abuse

◆ Reactions to prescribed medications

But now that more experts understand CFS and it is being seen as an individual disease process, it's more accepted that a person can, unfortunately, have a disease such as cancer or hypothyroidism and also have CFS. There is a lot of gray area within the diagnosis of CFS—for example, it can be both caused and worsened by conditions such as eating disorders.

In The Know

"More than half of our patients with Fibromyalgia Syndrome or Chronic Fatigue Syndrome develop a disordered pattern of breathing. They take very small, rapid breaths using the small muscles of their chest instead of slow, deep breathing with the large muscles of the abdomen. These changes are subtle and most people who 'hyper-ventilate' in this manner don't realize that their breathing pattern is out-of-synch.

Shallow chest breathing makes people feel tense. Slow, deep abdominal breathing creates feelings of calmness. Disordered breathing can also cause a broad array of frightening symptoms including mental fog, dizziness, irritability, chest pain, feeling numb, and more. Worsening symptoms then disrupt breathing further."

—*Richard Podell, M.D., Clinical Professor Robert Wood Johnson Medical School, New Jersey. CFS and FMS specialist.*

Fibromyalgia Syndrome

Fibromyalgia Syndrome (FMS) is a disorder that can be on the same continuum of CFS in that it causes fatigue, but there is more muscle pain than in CFS. People with FMS have classic and diagnostic "tender points" in specific places on the neck, shoulders, back, hips, arms, and legs. These tender points hurt when pressure is applied to them.

FMS also has symptoms of insomnia, morning stiffness, headaches, painful menstrual periods, numbness and tingling in the hands and feet, and brain fog that is distinc-tively called fibro-fog.

Although the causes of FMS are not known, it's believed to be linked to stress and traumatic events including such things as car accidents, illnesses, repetitive injuries, and certain diseases. FMS also can occur seemingly on its own. People who have rheumatoid arthritis, systemic lupus erythematosus (lupus), and ankylosing spondylitis (spinal arthritis) might be more likely to have FMS, too.

Although there is no defined treatment or medication to cure FMS, many family physicians, general internists, rheumatologists, physical therapists, and pain or rheu-matology clinics can help treat the symptoms of FMS. For more in-depth reading on fibromyalgia, check out *The Complete Idiot's Guide to Fibromyalgia.*

Adrenal Fatigue

Adrenal Fatigue Syndrome (AFS) is not an accepted medical diagnosis. Although it's not a recognized disorder, its symptoms occur with a high incidence in the general population. Like CFS in the past, people might often not be believed by their doctors and made to feel like hypochondriacs, although there are some doctors who do diagnose and treat AFS. This disorder is generally thought to be the result of extreme stress that overworks the adrenal glands—the glands responsible for the stress response in the body. When the adrenal glands become fatigued, they do not supply the body with adequate stress hormones and varying symptoms result.

The adrenal glands have a role in converting carbohydrate, protein, and fat to blood glucose for energy, fluid and electrolyte balance, immune function, and fat storage.

Generally, the symptoms of adrenal fatigue include fatigue; lethargy; and decreased energy in the mornings and between the hours of 3 P.M. and 5 P.M., when you typically self-medicate with some sort of stimulant such as coffee, soda, sugar, or salty foods.

Symptoms also can include the following:

- Light-headedness
- Feeling dizzy
- Fainting when rising from a sitting or reclined position
- Lowered blood pressure and blood sugar
- Brain fog
- Feeling generally unwell
- Hair loss
- Nausea
- Constipation and diarrhea
- Mild depression
- Insomnia
- Decreased libido
- Pain

- ◆ Increased symptoms of PMS

- ◆ Weight gain, particularly around the midsection

- ◆ Frequent flulike illnesses

Slip-Ups

If you have an invisible illness such as CFS, FMS, AFS, or even MS, chances are people won't see you as being sick. Instead of internalizing frustration when people tell you, "But you look so good!" verbalize or think something like, "Someday I plan to feel as well as I look." This will prevent you from opening yourself up to damage from negative stress while giving you the benefit of positive affirmations.

Most doctors will look only for extreme adrenal malfunction in the way of Addison's disease (when the glands produce markedly decreased cortisol) or Cushing's syndrome (excessive cortisol production) by testing adrenocorticotropic hormone (ACTH) levels and using a bell curve to identify abnormal levels. Doctors consider only the bottom and top 2 percent of the curve to be abnormal, so if your symptoms are 15 or 20 percent away from the mean (average), you might still be considered in the normal range.

Although you might never be officially diagnosed, you still can recover your life. Experts on adrenal fatigue agree that if it's severe, your recovery can take up to five years (most cases take one to two years). They also agree that using the measures outlined in this book to reduce fatigue stressors and improve positive thinking, as well as enjoying life, is the best treatment.

Gulf War Syndrome

Some armed services personnel who served during the Persian Gulf War in 1991 have been afflicted with a condition commonly known as Gulf War Syndrome. Though not validated by the U.S. government or the CDC, the constellation of symptoms includes fatigue, muscle and joint pain, headache, memory disturbances, and skin rash, among others. The CDC and other government agencies including the National Institutes of Health have, however, been conducting ongoing studies of the health impacts of chemical exposures during the Gulf War.

The syndrome seems to have a neurological base that many believe is linked to neurotoxin exposure during the war, including the nerve gas sarin, the anti-nerve gas drug pyridostigmine bromide, and neurotoxic pesticides. Many studies have taken place over the years showing that combat experience, psychiatric illness, or other deployment-related stressors don't account for the majority of symptoms experienced by Gulf War veterans.

Since March of 1999, there has been an ongoing National Center for Environmental Health (NCEH) study of other coalition troops, including the health status of Saudi Arabia National Guard troops to gather data on the adverse health effects of people who served in that region during that period of time. Other studies have shown that veterans deployed in the Persian Gulf War have a significantly higher incidence of chronic multisymptom illness.

Medical Treatments

Eating the Standard American Diet (SAD); exposure to environmental toxins; the use of alcohol; and the use of street drugs, over-the-counter (OTC), and prescription medicines can take a toll on your liver function—and the function of all your body systems, for that matter. Whether you take OTC medications or prescriptions, many drugs can cause you to have a generalized weakness and fatigue.

Although drugs do have definite benefits, the truth is all medications add foreign stuff to your body and all, even OTC drugs, have side effects. The effects of one drug's side effects can compound the next. If you are taking more than one drug at the same time, they can interact with one another. Even taken alone, the following medications can cause weakness or fatigue:

- Antianxiety medicines
- OTC and prescription antihistamines
- High blood pressure medicines
- Diuretics
- Prescription pain medicine
- Steroids
- Tricyclic antidepressants
- Statins

Talk to your doctor about your medications or the combinations you are taking if you feel they are causing or adding to your fatigue.

Chemotherapy

Fatigue caused by cancer treatment can be similar to that of CFS. This sort of chemotherapy-induced chronic fatigue isn't improved with rest or sleep and can last for weeks, months, and in some cases years after treatment. Fortunately, most people regain their energy after six months to a year, but those with more intensive treatment including stem cell or bone marrow transplant might have to deal with fatigue for a much longer period of time.

Cancer fatigue affects nearly everyone who has chemotherapy and is the most common and, most say, most distressing side effect. The fatigue also can be caused by anemia that accompanies some cancers and some treatments. Your red blood cells carry oxygen to your cells, and when you don't have enough of them, you don't get the oxygen you need so you end up with shortness of breath, weariness, and lack of energy.

In The Know
Although fatigue looks like depression in cancer or hepatitis treatment, it's entirely possible to be fatigued but not depressed. Sorting out the two can include looking closely at whether you lack the ability to feel pleasure or have feelings of sadness, hopelessness, despair, or guilt that are typical of depression and not of fatigue. While medical treatments including radiation can cause such fatigue that you cannot care for your hygiene or other activities of daily living, if you are more distressed about not being able to perform basic daily activities than not having any interest in doing them at all, it's more likely you are being affected by fatigue and not depression.

After years of chemotherapy patients complaining about continual brain fog and fatigue post treatment, researchers have finally found that chemotherapy does cause changes to the brain's metabolism and blood flow. These changes, dubbed *chemo brain*, can linger for as long as ten years after a person has chemotherapy, and include the inability to focus or multitask and poor memory.

Hepatitis Treatment

It's not just cancer chemotherapy that can have lasting adverse effects, but the treatment for chronic hepatitis using such drugs as pegylated interferon and ribaviron also is being shown to cause a lasting posttreatment syndrome that is similar to CFS in some people.

Although the drugs are known to be neurotoxic (brain poison) and can cause extreme fatigue and chemotherapy-like side effects during treatment, they have not been widely acknowledged to cause long-lasting brain effects. Because the treatments are so new, there have not been studies as to the incidents of posttreatment syndrome, although there are many anecdotal reports. Today, most doctors who administer this treatment will admit that it can take a year or longer to recover from this CFS-like posttreatment syndrome.

Energy Bar _____

If you are taking chemotherapy or any neurotoxic medical treatment, be sure to eat a lot of brain foods rich in omega-3 fatty acids, B vitamins, choline, antioxidants, and beta-carotene. Foods to look for include salmon, yellowfin tuna, mackerel, sardines, beef liver, eggs, peanut butter, spinach, cranberries, sweet potatoes, strawberries, kidney beans, raisin bran (made without added sugar), lamb loin, and wheat germ.

Radiation

Radiation therapy can cause fatigue that increases over time, and as the treatment continues. It might last from a few months to a year or longer after treatment ends, particularly for people who are receiving bone marrow transplants.

HIV/AIDS

Fatigue is a recognized symptom of HIV infection and AIDS that affects a person's quality of life, her treatment, and even her long-term outcome. And often during the very initial acute stage of HIV infection, fatigue is a common symptom. It can have a combination of causes including anemia, lung function impairment, and hormonal and nutritional deficiencies. Like cancer chemotherapy, anemia is the most common cause of fatigue in people with HIV/AIDS and is sometimes caused by the common antiviral agent zidovudine, opportunistic infections, and nutritional deficiencies.

Depression contributes to fatigue in people living with HIV/AIDS. Continually dealing with a progressive disability or a chronic terminal illness, the stress of work, stigmatization, social isolation, and opportunistic infections and malignancies that sometimes cause changes in the brain are all factors that can cause depression, inactivity, and insomnia—which can all contribute to fatigue.

The Least You Need to Know

◆ Fatigue is a major symptom of multiple sclerosis (MS), cancer, hepatitis B and C, HIV and AIDS, and the treatments for them.

◆ Chronic Fatigue Syndrome (CFS) is a complex and debilitating illness that is primarily characterized by profound fatigue that doesn't improve with rest or sleep, with other symptoms including brain fog, weakness, pain, alcohol intolerance, night sweats, depression, weight loss, and many other symptoms.

◆ Fibromyalgia syndrome (FMS) is a disorder that can be on the same continuum of CFS in that it causes fatigue, but there is more muscle pain than in CFS characterized by classic and diagnostic "tender points" on specific places on the neck, shoulders, back, hips, arms, and legs.

◆ Adrenal Fatigue Syndrome (AFS) and Gulf War Syndrome are not accepted medical diagnoses, but some researchers believe they may be the cause of severe symptoms including fatigue.

◆ Whether you take OTC medications or prescriptions, many drugs can cause you to have a generalized weakness and fatigue.

4

Lifestyle Causes

In This Chapter

◆ Why to say no to junk and processed food

◆ Stimulants can get you in deeper

◆ Watch out for brain poisons

◆ How addictions worsen fatigue

◆ Excessive behaviors are as harmful as drugs

◆ Shift work and chronic fatigue

Unhealthy lifestyles are a major contributing factor to general unwellness and even serious illness. In fact weeding out and correcting poor lifestyle habits are the meat of the interventions laid out in this book. Taking personal responsibility and learning how to make the right choices will have the biggest impact on your wellness now and help you secure a healthy future.

It's a fact that today the United States can no longer pride itself on being a nation of healthy people full of vitality. The medical community now direly predicts that children today will not outlive their parents due to obesity, toxicity, and the lack of nutrients in the Standard American Diet (SAD).

Fatigue is a red flag waving at you. You need to surrender all your fatigue stressors, including your diet of processed food. Other lifestyle factors such as extreme behaviors are also within your control. Correcting them will help to protect you against fatigue and other health problems. You can also learn how certain behaviors, habits, addictions, and factors like shift work can result in chronic fatigue and decrease your overall quality of life. Remember this chapter just clues you into your lifestyle—keep reading because subsequent chapters will explain steps you can take to maintain a healthy way of life.

Diet

Eating a proper diet of real whole food requires knowing how to put meals together, and that means buying real food and preparing or cooking it! But many people simply don't know how to cook because they didn't have moms and grandmas who cooked or because they do not have the time or do not take the time to do it. Unfortunately, even if you do cook, creating meals with recipes that use processed ingredients isn't any better than eating fast food or restaurant fare.

If you've grown up on a diet of convenient processed foods and are unaware of the lack of nutrients and added toxins in your food, making the connection from your diet to your health problems—such as fatigue—might be a stretch. But, know that a poor diet is one of the major causes, and thankfully one of the easiest fixes, of chronic fatigue.

Junk, Processed, and Restaurant Food

Even though everyone is eating processed food, is it really okay? Processed food is truly convenient, it requires little or no preparation, it's relatively cheap, and it usually tastes wildly good. It comes out of a package, can, or box and doesn't spoil or rot like fresh food does. In fact, some products will stay preserved for years if unopened. That's a lot of pros in the argument for eating a diet of processed food. So what's the catch?

First, there's no recommended daily allowance (RDA) for the hundreds of chemical ingredients in processed food. They're just there to color, stabilize, soften, emulsify, sweeten, bleach, improve texture, preserve, scent, and flavor. But your body doesn't recognize those additives as food or any other element it requires. Salt (sodium chloride) is added to most processed foods to prevent spoiling, add flavor, thicken, reduce dryness, increase sweetness, and disguise metallic or chemical aftertastes. Salt also helps to create an addiction and craving for some processed foods. Even though it's a good and necessary mineral in your diet, it's overprevalent in a diet of processed foods. This causes high blood pressure, which complicates diabetes, and is a major cause of heart disease and stroke.

Some food labels carry endorsements that are designed to inspire your confidence. But here's the deal. You know how every so often consumers get blasted by the media with warnings about certain food groups to avoid or to limit in our diet? "Stay away from fat, especially the saturated kind." "Eat low-carb." "Avoid sugar; use the man-made chemical stuff instead." And one of the most preposterous warnings, "Don't eat eggs (real food)." With each new recommendation, consumers get more and more confused. As you will find out in Chapter 10, a diet of real whole food eliminates the guesswork because whole food is naturally designed to be healthy whereas manufactured food is designed for reasons including long shelf life and convenience.

Trans fats are on the top of the list of evil fats because they aren't good for you in any amount and your body has zero requirements for them. *Trans fatty acids* raise your bad cholesterol (LDL) and lower your good cholesterol (HDL). Some, not all, trans fat has been removed from packaged foods and some fast food. But until chemists can come up with another way of keeping food products fresh and crispy, trans fats are bound to remain in products. The point is that you simply cannot trust laboratory and man-made food products and additives because when and if trans fat is avoided completely, other questionable lab creations will likely replace it.

def•i•ni•tion

Tiny amounts of natural **trans fat** occur in beef and dairy foods. However, the more common artificial trans fats are created when hydrogen gas reacts with oil to make partially hydrogenated vegetable oil. Hydrogenated vegetable oil, high in **trans fatty acids,** is the oil that's in the majority of processed food and is used to extend shelf life and create desirable mouth feels, like crispiness.

The trans fat in cookies, crackers, potato chips, icing, margarine, and microwave popcorn has been found to be a factor in obesity and clogged arteries, virtually doubling your risk of heart attack and increasing your risk of stroke.

The base of most processed food is refined corn, soybeans, wheat, and rice. Grain (seed) is cheap. It's cheap to feed to animals, it's cheap to process, and it stores easily. These grains are used to create wildly unhealthy refined carbs and test-tube sugars such as high fructose corn syrup. Both of these cause your blood sugar to rapidly spike while providing too many calories.

Oils manufactured from grain seeds, including sunflower, safflower, corn, cottonseed, and soybean oils, are high in the essential fatty acid omega-6 and are ubiquitous in processed foods.

You need a balance of the fatty acids, but a diet of processed, refined, junk, and manufactured food gives you too much omega-6 and not enough omega-3. It's thought that this imbalance might be the source of the rise in conditions and diseases such as asthma, coronary heart disease, some forms of cancer, and autoimmune and neurodegenerative diseases that all have some link to inflammation in the body. Research points to this imbalance as adding to the crisis of obesity, dyslexia, depression, and hyperactivity in developed countries whose primary food source is manufactured, processed, and refined food.

So, you're laboriously reading labels as you've been told in an attempt to avoid or reduce ingredients that have been 86'd. But can you actually pronounce and do you really understand those hundreds of chemical ingredients on your food labels? The truth is that, although you feel you are making a conscious effort, following guidelines and reading labels on your very convenient quick-from-the-pantry-to-the-table meals, manufactured food just isn't in the same league nutrition-wise as the real thing. Your boxed breakfast or frozen entrée with its added and enriched made-in-test-tubes vitamins and massed-produced, low-end, cheap ingredients, doesn't compare with the real deal. That is, real whole food with its intrinsic components such as vitamin C and E, beta-carotene, and lycopene is much healthier.

It's pretty obvious that an apple, for example, is actually food. It's good for your health and doesn't need a labeled endorsement to tell you that. The many compounds intrinsic in real food work synergistically to nourish your body and to create hundreds of other elements you need. Those products that add a smidgen of what once was a fruit or vegetable are simply not going to give you the different compounds and elements you need daily.

Nutrients aside, processed food is also lifeless food because of its lack of beneficial enzymes and fibrous material. Processing does away with the natural fiber necessary for healthy digestion. It has resulted in an epidemic of constipation. When toxins are not excreted and food sits in your colon fermenting, it causes and adds to problems such as colon cancer, fatigue, irritable bowel syndrome, and allergies. Processing also destroys the enzymes in food that are necessary catalysts for internal chemical reactions, including healthy digestion. Without those enzymes from real whole food, your pancreas is strained to produce the enzymes your body needs and the result again is lowered resistance, immune system dysfunction, and degenerative diseases, including cancer and chronic fatigue.

In The Know

The brain is made of fats and oils. When people flood their diets with seed oils and omega-6 fatty acids, it forces out the omega-3s and the neurons. Instead of looking like full, healthy trees with wonderful branches and leaves, the synapses become rather shriveled and die back. The result [he says] can be depression, suicidal thoughts, and even criminal behavior. Some of that is controversial. But a committee established by the American Psychiatric Association did recommend that doctors consider omega-3 supplements as part of the treatment for depression.

—Dr. Sanjay Gupta, CNN "Fed Up, America's Killer Diet"

So, let's add up all the cons of processed food:

◆ It lacks the essential synergist compounds intrinsic in real food.

◆ It contains test-tube sugars like high fructose corn syrup and refined carbs that cause rapid and unhealthy spikes in your blood sugar and provides too many calories.

◆ It contains exorbitant, unhealthy amounts of salt; oodles of health-killing trans fats; and loads of chemicals that are added in small FDA-approved amounts that, when eaten as a steady diet, add up to a toxic load.

Processed food gives your body a double whammy. While providing an insufficient amount of nutrients, it places undue stress on your body.

Coffee and Stimulants

Caffeine is a legal, over-the-counter (OTC), central nervous system stimulant that does a number on many systems. It increases gastric secretion (heartburn), worsens insulin sensitivity, and alters your blood pH balance causing acidity, all of which are factors in the development of inflammatory diseases and cancer.

Caffeine provides a short-term boost by stimulating the release of the hormones norepinephrine, dopamine, and adrenaline that are released by adrenal glands in times of stress (flight or fight mode), causing your blood sugar to spike. And what goes up also comes down, so attempt after attempt to falsely boost your energy eventually fails when the energy banks of your body are depleted and stimulants lose their effect. The caffeine-induced overstimulation of the nervous system also can increase feelings of anxiety and make sleeping difficult. So as your sleep debt increases, so does your intake of stimulants.

Caffeine causes what researchers at Johns Hopkins University call "caffeine dependence syndrome," described as having three of the following four criteria:

◆ Withdrawal symptoms including headache, fatigue, and depression

◆ Caffeine consumption that continues even with the awareness of the psychological or physical problems it's causing, such as worsening an ulcer or insomnia

◆ Attempted but unsuccessful efforts to cut back on caffeine

◆ Caffeine tolerance such as the ability to drink a cup of coffee and still fall asleep

There are plenty of studies released in an attempt to soothe your mind about drinking coffee. Are the coffee-addicted researchers only attempting to reassure themselves? Or are researchers like Dr. Thomas Perls, a longevity expert, correct when he tells us, "More than two cups of coffee a day will trim life expectancy by a year or more."

Slip-Ups

Stimulants don't create energy like sleep, good nutrition, and stress reduction do. They only create false energy while forcing your body to use up stored energy. Depending on false energy from stimulant use can result in a state of chronic fatigue.

Could this be because caffeine puts your body in a state of chronic stress, spikes blood sugar, and depletes important vitamins such as B-complex vitamins and vitamin C? Chronic use of caffeine causes and worsens the same symptoms that it's used to soothe, including fatigue, headache, moodiness, and even depression.

Sugar is another legal stimulant and is a socially accepted addictive substance that is hidden in all processed foods from salad dressing to pizza. In addition, you simply cannot go out to eat at most restaurants without inadvertently consuming sugar in some form; typically high fructose corn syrup.

Sugar fed to lab rats causes dependence in as little as ten days with withdrawal symptoms including anxiety, chattering teeth, and tremors—the same symptoms seen in withdrawal from drugs. This study extrapolated to humans illustrates that once addicted, a little sugar isn't enough. Instead, just a taste can send an addicted person into a tailspin binge. Sugar causes a temporary energy lift because it's quickly metabolized into the bloodstream. For this reason, it also raises your insulin level too high and too fast while inhibiting the release of growth hormones, depressing your immune system; and opening you up to all kinds of illness including the recent epidemic of autoimmune and degenerative diseases. High glucose levels cause inflammation, which underlies such problems as arthritis, immune system dysfunction, and autoimmune diseases (not to mention facial wrinkles!).

Other quick fixes people might use in an effort to combat fatigue include illegal drugs such as cocaine and over-the-counter supplements that often contain dangerous stimulants such as ephedra (Ma Huang) and guarana. Most products that claim to be remedies for fatigue just contain extraordinarily high levels of caffeine that can cause rapid, abnormal heart rhythms, heart attack, and—depending on your health—even death. The downside of all stimulants is the revolving door of fatigue, tolerance, and dependence on the substance.

Brain Poisons

Because most of what are considered *brain poisons* are surrounded by considerable controversy and vigorous debate, it's up to your own personal investigation to choose to avoid them or not. These substances are allowed in food most likely because the toxic effects of certain brain poisons are so insidious and that major damage often takes years to produce observable clinical effects on behavior, memory, and learning. Like sorting out all the potential causes of fatigue, deciding whether brain poisons are affecting you can take some effort and dedication on your part.

Some food additives and elements also can have the effect of being slow and subtle poisons to your brain and nervous system (neurotoxins). Certain potential brain poisons that researchers have looked at include *aspartame, sucralose, monosodium glutamate (MSG)*, artificial *food colors*, and *mercury*. According to Dr. Blaylock, a board-certified neurosurgeon, lecturer, and author of the book, *Excitotoxins: The Taste That Kills*, food additives, including MSG, aspartame, and L-cysteine known by researchers as "exitotoxins" have brain toxic effects.

def•i•ni•tion

Brain poisons are neurotoxic substances that cause damage to nerves or nerve tissues. **MSG, aspartame, sucralose, mercury,** and **food colorings** are a group known by some researchers as "slow neurotoxins" that, after prolonged exposure, can result in neurodegenerative diseases. Some brain poisons also can cause acute symptoms in some people.

Mercury is a brain poison found both in contaminated fish and in dental (amalgam) fillings. Mercury has been linked to brain, kidney, and immune system damage; gastrointestinal problems; sleep disturbances; concentration and memory disturbances; apathy; restlessness; Alzheimer's disease; bleeding gums; and other disorders.

Large cold-water fish have had the most exposure to mercury-polluted waters, so they carry the highest risk of mercury contamination. The FDA has recommended that pregnant women, breastfeeding mothers, and young children avoid eating fish such as shark, swordfish, tilefish, king mackerel, and fresh and frozen tuna. For other adults, regular consumption of fish should be limited to about seven ounces per week. Your best bet is to ask at your fish counter when you buy fish. The safest fish are usually listed there along with current warnings.

Dental amalgams are another controversial topic and believed by some to be the source of some instances of fibromyalgia, chronic fatigue, anorexia, and recurrent depression. Ever since amalgams first came into use in dentistry, there has been discussion and debate as to whether they release mercury and other toxic metals into the body.

Aspartame is a chemical sweetener believed by many to be a brain poison that accounts for a huge percentage of the adverse reactions related to food additives that are reported to the FDA. These reactions include headaches, anxiety attacks, arthritis, asthma, brain cancer, chronic fatigue, depression, insomnia, memory loss, migraines, numbness of extremities, seizures, tachycardia, tinnitus, vertigo, vision loss, and—astonishingly enough—even weight gain due to the cravings it causes. Whew! It's also thought that some chronic illnesses can be worsened or even caused by ingesting aspartame, including multiple sclerosis, epilepsy, Chronic Fatigue Syndrome (CFS), Parkinson's disease, Alzheimer's disease, fibromyalgia, and diabetes.

Sucralose is an artificial sweetener made by replacing some molecules on sugar with chlorine. Although sucralose manufacturers want to convince you that sucralose is like sugar because it's made from sugar, it in fact is a chemical made in a test tube. Sucralose is not completely eliminated from your body when ingested but is absorbed in small amounts and distributed to essentially all tissues. Like aspartame, many adverse effects of sucralose have been reported to the FDA, including migraines and even seizures. Artificial sweeteners only increase your cravings for sweets and carbs, but cutting back on processed foods and eating real food puts you ahead in the game by also reducing your craving for sweets.

MSG is a well-known brain poison that used to be a common seasoning in Chinese food. MSG was found to cause what became known as Chinese restaurant syndrome, a constellation of symptoms: headache, flushing, sweating, a sensation of pressure in the mouth or face, chest pain, and shortness of breath. Because this "hidden" brain poison is a common ingredient in just about all processed foods, symptoms of headaches, stomach disorders, fatigue, depression, food cravings, and many other problems might in fact be caused or exacerbated by the ingestion of MSG.

Slip-Ups

Although most people are aware of the adverse effects of MSG, they don't know that MSG is a hidden additive listed on food labels as hydrolyzed vegetable protein, hydrolyzed protein, hydrolyzed plant protein, plant protein extract, sodium caseinate, calcium caseinate, yeast extract, textured protein, autolyzed yeast, and hydrolyzed oat flour. It may also be known as malt extract, malt flavoring, bouillon, broth, stock, flavoring, natural flavoring, carrageenan, enzymes, soy protein concentrate, soy protein isolate, and whey protein concentrate.

Although manufactured food is still synthesized from mostly real food and not synthetic compounds like petroleum, it does contain petroleum, acetone, and coal-tar–based ingredients such as artificial colors and dyes that are widely used to alter the appearance of foods, drugs, and cosmetics. Similar to all additives, the safety of food coloring is determined by studies that aim to assess the risk of death that is caused by a substance. The lower the chance that a substance is lethal, the more we are supposed to be assured that a substance is safe.

Because FD & C Red No. 2 dye was shown to produce cancer in experimental animals, the dye was removed from general use. But most studies are not even looking for the subtle, insidious symptoms or effects on behavior, personality, and learning ability or other neurological damaging effects additives are having on humans after prolonged use.

Moms have great powers of observation and very often perform their own informal studies within their families, finding that food additives cause behaviors similar to attention deficit disorder or hyperactivity and allergies in their kids. They then remove those additives from their diet. If you add up a day's worth of food coloring intake from all sources, it might concern you to realize that the amount of petroleum, acetone, and coal-tar–based substances you are consuming. This source of potential brain poison can be adding to your symptoms of fatigue.

Although controversy and debate still rage and studies are still ongoing in regard to some of these so-called safe but possibly neurotoxic agents, it might be worth performing your own personal research study by removing these potential brain poisons from your diet.

Slip-Ups

Soda and other colored and artificially flavored beverages are terrible offenders and causes of chronic fatigue because they contain massive amounts of sugar or aspartame, and all of them contain petroleum-based dyes.

Chances are that by removing mercury fillings in your teeth and additives like MSG, aspartame, and petroleum and other chemical-based products from your food, you just might improve your allergies, GI problems, and other symptoms (including your fatigue). Remember your mom asking you, "If everyone else jumped off a bridge, would you jump too?" That might be helpful to consider when you are trying to decide whether to ingest additives and other chemical ingredients that are in your processed foods and beverages.

Addictions: Smoking, Alcohol, and Drugs

Nicotine and alcohol are two of the most common causes of fatigue. If you've been smoking for many years and weren't previously bothered by fatigue, you might not attribute your fatigue to smoking. But cigarette smoke pollutes your oxygen supply with toxic compounds such as carbon monoxide. The buildup of these toxins over time can cause and contribute to fatigue. Because nicotine is a stimulant, as you quit smoking, the withdrawal symptoms can cause a sense of temporary fatigue. Nicotine withdrawal also interferes with falling asleep and can cause waking during the night that will add to your fatigue.

Although many people self-medicate with alcohol in an attempt to wind down for sleep, it has been found that alcohol consumption disrupts the second half of the sleep cycle and causes awakening and difficulty getting back to sleep. The disruption in sleep then leads to fatigue and sleepiness. Alcohol also increases toxic buildup and acts as a nervous depressant, thus causing fatigue.

Fatigue is also a side effect of many prescription and OTC medications, including antihistamines. Dependency on or abuse of street drugs and alcohol often goes hand in hand with chronic fatigue. In addition, fatigue is often the culprit when you recently start, stop, or change medicines. Withdrawal from drugs, alcohol, and nicotine all can produce depression, fatigue, and headache. Thus, it can be helpful to keep a record of what you took the night before when you wake up fatigued.

Workaholism

If your need to work is out of balance with normal living, you might have an obsessive-compulsive disorder known as workaholism. In other words, work is your drug of choice. Workaholics are out of balance because, even away from work, they are unable to turn it off (for example, talking about work while supposedly on vacation). This is thought to be due to factors such as not wanting to deal with relationships and an internal desire to escape intimacy.

Workaholics get their high from putting in long hours to mask anxiety about other areas of their lives that they are ignoring. But workaholism creates other difficulties such as family problems and ironically reduced, not increased, productivity. Because the minds and bodies of workaholics are not adequately rested, they frequently have outbursts of temper and are irritable, impatient, and restless. Workaholics are prone to insomnia and an inability to relax. They are forgetful, have difficulty concentrating, and experience boredom and mood swings (euphoria to depression). This overwork drug also causes symptoms of headaches, fatigue, indigestion, chest pain, shortness of breath, nervous tics, and dizziness.

Workaholics aren't generally known to have the ability to delegate authority or tasks, and they aren't team players because they feel that everything is all about them. At the same time, they ignore other important aspects of their lives, including family and relationships. You don't have to work outside the home to be a workaholic. Workaholics can be anyone from women who stay home to be 100 percent devoted to their kids to anyone in any job or profession who works to the exclusion of proper rest and relaxation, stress reduction, diet, exercise, fun, and fostering relationships.

Perfectionism

Perfectionists have unrealistically high standards and expectations, are highly critical of their own and other's performance, and typically have a compulsion toward impossible goals. Their self-worth depends on high levels of achievement. Studies have shown that perfectionists tend to be fatigued, irritable, and discouraged. They continually produce higher amounts of stress hormones such as cortisol because of their constant internal pressures. Their feelings of anger, fatigue, excitability, and cognitive impairment caused by continual stress increase their risk for health problems.

Perfectionists are not the most efficient people because they often have to go over the same task again and again before they can go on to the next one. Their need for excellence, together with their fear of failure, puts them on a collision course of continual stress. Perfectionism often goes hand in hand with other destructive compulsions like overexercising and eating disorders (the need for a perfect body), workaholism (the need for unrealistic work-related achievement), and other addictive behaviors. Because a person is experiencing the sum of a number of continual stressors on her mind and body, the result is often depression, anger, hostility, impatience, anxiety, and fatigue.

Overexercise

There is no bigger head trip than that experienced by an overexerciser when he becomes too fatigued to work out. Those who overexercise tend to equate health with fitness in extreme ways. They falsely believe that the levels of extreme exercise are benefiting their bodies when in fact overexercise has long-term health consequences. So, when they reach a point of fatigue that limits or prevents exercise, they cannot understand what is wrong.

Compulsive exercise also is called obligatory exercise, anorexia athletica, and exercise bulimia. Although most people begin exercising with fitness or fun in mind, when taken to extremes, it becomes an addiction. If you have reached a point where you feel compelled to exercise and experience guilt and anxiety when you are not able to, you have a problem. When you plan your life around exercise and exercise even if you're injured or ill, in bad weather, and in place of social activities, it's a compulsion and it's time to seek help.

Compulsive exercise is often used by people to feel more in control of their lives, to define their self-worth, and to help them cope with low self-esteem. Working out every day is not necessarily a compulsion, but if you are hammered with feelings of defeat and despair because you can't work out for any reason, that's a problem. This compulsion can cause physical and psychological harm, including anxiety and depression and damage to tendons, ligaments, bones, cartilage, and joints—particularly when you don't give minor injuries time to heal. Too much exercise doesn't build; it destroys muscle mass, especially if you aren't getting proper nutrition. Excessive exercise in women sometimes disrupts the menstrual cycle, which can also lead to premature bone loss (osteoporosis). And working out excessively eventually leads to exhaustion and chronic fatigue.

Chronic fatigue in a compulsive exerciser is a major indication that you need to stop all exercise. Get professional help to stop and to manage your feelings if you need to. Then resume a balanced and healthy program along with a reduction of all other fatigue stressors in your life only after you have fully recovered from your fatigue. If you don't, you might find yourself out of commission permanently. Compulsive exercise coupled with other extreme fatigue stressors can and does lead many to experience CFS.

Lack of Exercise

Acute fatigue is usually related to factors such as lack of exercise. If you're too tired to exercise, you might decide to skip it, but then when you do work out, you might end up getting tired more easily because you're out of shape. This might set you up to be discouraged so start slow whenever you're deconditioned.

Exercise boosts the release of endorphins so you experience less pain. It also increases your level of serotonin, which works to improve your mood and make blood vessels flexible thereby reducing pain. Serotonin helps to regulate healthy sleep cycles. Lack of exercise then feeds into depressive moods, pain, and insomnia. Additionally, deconditioned and atrophied muscles tend to spasm, causing and increasing pain and interfering with sleep.

Energy Bar

Plan to get moderate physical activity for at least a half-hour on most days of the week to improve your fatigue and mood and to decrease stress. One reason exercise actually improves sleep is because it causes you to be physically tired enough to sleep.

Shift Work

If you work the night shift, chances are you suffer from Shift Work Sleep Disorder (SWSD). Working during the night forces your body to function outside of your natural circadian rhythm. Because morning sunlight signals to your brain that it's time to wake up, people with SWSD live in a constant state of circadian disruption and sleep deprivation.

When your circadian rhythms are disrupted regularly, you body can't rest and rebuild as it needs to. People with SWSD have symptoms such as fatigue, insomnia, disrupted sleep schedule, problems with personal relationships, irritability, depression, reduced performance, and sleepiness at work. Because so much of the general population works off-hour shifts, it's estimated that up to 5 percent of the workforce suffers from SWSD. If you are a shift worker, answering yes to the following questions can indicate that you have SWSD:

◆ Are you overly tired and fatigued but have trouble sleeping?

◆ Have your work-related sleep problems persisted for at least one month?

◆ Is your fatigue problem affecting your social, family, or work life?

Natalie was 35 years old when she first became fatigued. As a nurse and single mom of a 5-year-old boy, Natalie had many strikes against her. While she considered herself an athlete and hardworking, Natalie had extreme and toxic behaviors that ended her career and her life as she knew it when she developed full blown CFS at age 39 after years of ignoring symptoms. So where did Natalie do wrong?

Natalie's diet was mostly prepared from processed ingredients or restaurant meals. At 5' 5" tall, she weighed 110 pounds and prided herself on her extreme exercise accomplishments, often working out after a night shift on little to no sleep. Coffee, sugar, and diet sodas were part of her everyday diet. She was underweight and undernourished for her extreme exercise behavior and worked for many years with Shift Work Sleep Disorder and chronic exhaustion. Natalie came into work early, stayed late, and volunteered regularly for extra shifts even when feeling exhausted. And, to top it off, she was a closet smoker.

While you may not feel as out of balance as Natalie seems to have been, if you are fatigued it's important to add up all your own fatigue stressors in order to look at how they may be compounding each other. Fatigue is your body's way of telling you that something is wrong.

The Least You Need to Know

- Poor diet is the most common but easily fixed cause of fatigue.

- Stimulants like caffeine, nicotine, sugar, ephedra, guarana, and some street drugs are used by many as a pick-me-up. But chronic and excessive use of stimulants leads to tolerance, dependence, addiction, and increased fatigue.

- Brain poisons are used as additives and allowed in FDA-approved amounts in foods. Mercury is a brain poison found in cold-water fish and dental amalgams. Although controversial, it's worth taking the effort to investigate whether brain poisons such as mercury; aspartame; sucralose; MSG; and dyes used to color food, drugs, and cosmetics are factoring into your fatigue.

- Drug use, alcohol consumption, and smoking all have cumulative effects that cause or lead to chronic fatigue.

- Workaholism, perfectionism, and compulsive exercise are used to self-medicate, and all have toxic repercussions on your personal life, work life, and physical and mental health.

- People who work outside the normal nine-to-five work hours can suffer from Shift Work Sleep Disorder and live in a constant state of circadian disruption and sleep deprivation.

5

Psychological Causes

In This Chapter

- ◆ The fallout of stress and burnout
- ◆ Anxiety and depression could be the cause
- ◆ Is it depression or CFS?
- ◆ How emotions take their toll
- ◆ The impact of drugs, legal or not

There are literally hundreds of diseases that cause fatigue, but even so, of all the people who see a doctor for fatigue, less than 10 percent actually have a medical condition or disease. Given those odds, and because fatigue is a major symptom of many psychiatric disorders, it's likely your doctor may consider a psychological cause—particularly if you check out medically.

The way doctors work is that they first look at the physical and then the psychological, and all while considering social causes. Still, they are not likely to closely analyze the cumulative effect of all stressors on your life to see the causes of your fatigue and the breadth of the physical and psychosocial dimensions of all your fatigue stressors.

I know you're feeling whipped, but because the bigger picture is not always clear when it comes to sorting out the many causes, this chapter will help you to determine whether your fatigue does have a psychological component.

You might be able to connect more dots as you try to determine whether your fatigue is entirely psychological or is being fueled by some of the other fatigue stressors discussed in this book.

Stress and Burnout

The adrenal glands are the small, triangular-shaped glands located on the top of the kidneys whose job is to prepare the body during times of stress for fight-or-flight with the release of "stress" hormones including adrenaline, noradrenaline, and cortisol. When this stress response is activated, your blood, pulse, and blood sugar level increase; blood is shunted away from your digestive system to vital fighting organs like your brain and heart; your pupils dilate; and the speed of your reflexes increases, all for the purpose of survival.

In these modern times we aren't being hunted by lions and tigers, but we still have the same fight-or-flight reaction during physical, emotional, or mental stress. That means if you live in a state of constant stress, it will, over time, impact the way your adrenal glands function and lead to fatigue, illness (including heart disease and cancer), and physical and mental burnout. Continual stress is internal wear and tear, folks.

Your body interprets all stress and pressures as a threat to your life. When you add other fatigue stressors such as inadequate sleep and stimulants—including the less-obvious ones like exposure to excessive noise—you will find it even more difficult to cope with stress. For example, consider some continual stressors: a week of insufficient sleep or overwork, feelings of internal pressure or mental stress, and a poor diet. Add these up and you get a body that is in a state of constant activation of the stress response system, making you even more vulnerable to everyday pressures including mental health problems such as anxiety and depression. It also weakens your immune system function, setting you up to get sick. If you then encounter something like a flu bug and you continue pounding your systems with stress, you are circling the drain so to speak.

Energy Bar

Many studies show that individuals who exercise at least two to three times a week experience considerably less depression, anger, cynical distrust, and stress than those who exercise less often or not at all.

Burnout is a state of extreme emotional and physical exhaustion caused by prolonged and excessive stress. It typically comes from striving too hard without satisfaction in your job or other endeavors and is compounded by the fatigue stressors outlined in this book. Burnout can occur after feeling overwhelmed and unable to meet continual and constant demands. As the stressors continue, you then begin to lose any interest or motivation that first brought you to pursue a job or take on a role. The result is that your productivity drastically decreases and you feel fatigued, apathetic, increasingly powerless, hopeless, cynical, and resentful. Burnout can eventually threaten your job, your health, and your relationships.

Most people are aware of being under a lot of stress, but you might not always notice burnout when it happens. But it's roots are excessive stress and it's a gradual process, so watch for the red flags of burnout: feelings of being physically and emotionally drained, detachment, isolation, withdrawal (both at work and at home), feeling trapped, and feelings of failure. If you see a red flag waving, it's time to bail or get help.

Shift work and work that requires life-and-death decisions and actions typically lead to burnout. A nurse, a doctor, or anyone else working rotating shifts with money, lives, or community services on the line can be a prescription for burnout. Those people often have an internal nagging voice continually reminding them of the stressor that is pushing them into burnout. So, if you are one of them, never tell yourself that just because someone else is dealing with a certain stressor that you should be able to. Instead, look at it as something you must deal with and find a new job, work different hours, or even make a career move or change.

Like the expression "stressed out," the term "burned out" is thrown about by many people, but the true meaning of burnout is an intense physical, mental, and emotional response that can be crippling and devastating. Burnout can, in fact, lead to severe health problems including Chronic Fatigue Syndrome (CFS), addictions, and fatal errors at work. All of it, in turn, impacts lives even more severely when relationships crumble and careers and lifestyles are lost. John is a 30-year-old manager of a large courier company. As a salaried employee, he worked 12 to 14 hours a day 6 days a week over a period of many years. The only benefit from his job is a paycheck. John felt chronically tired, cynical, angry, and depressed. He experienced anxiety and frequent colds and flu. John knew he needed to either quit this job or reduce his hours, but was mentally and physically exhausted and unable to make decisions. Finally in a fit of anger, he told his boss that he had to cut his hours or quit. John is now enrolled in college classes, working less hours, and feeling healthier, more positive, and hopeful about his future.

By recognizing the early warning signs of severe stress, you can avoid burnout and subsequent overwhelming problems such as CFS. Be alert for signs of severe stress: problems sleeping; aches and pains; eating disorders; outbursts of emotions; high blood pressure; and GI problems like ulcers, stomach aches, and diarrhea.

You can have CFS-like symptoms if you are experiencing burnout related to your job or any other circumstance. But because those work-related, CFS-like illnesses are typically much shorter in duration, when you have severe symptoms that continue, your doctor should consider CFS as a diagnosis.

Depression

Depression is a very serious medical illness involving the brain. This disorder involves more than just feeling a little blue or down for a few days. It's a persistent feeling of sadness and hopelessness that interferes with everyday life.

Many symptoms are associated with major depression, but the most common are a continual depressed mood every day, considerable weight gain or loss (generally 10 percent or more), restlessness, low energy or tiredness every day, trouble sleeping or excessive sleeping, a sense of being slowed down, feelings of worthlessness or of guilt, an inability to concentrate and/or make decisions, and suicidal thoughts.

Depression typically begins between the ages of 15 and 30 and is more common in women than men. It sometimes runs in families or develops after the birth of a baby, as with postpartum depression. A lack of sunlight during the winter can cause seasonal affective disorder (SAD) resulting in depression. Depression is also one aspect of bipolar (manic-depressive) disorder.

Because fatigue is such a common symptom of depression, most doctors will consider it as a diagnosis if a medical workup is negative for any other disorder. Doctors consider fatigue to be unexplained (idiopathic) if they cannot give you a medical diagnosis. Because it's out of the scope of most doctors to consider all the fatigue stressors as causative factors, if they see severe fatigue along with a large number of unexplained complaints, they are more likely to give a diagnosis of depression. Doctors simply don't have time in the usual 15 minute office visit to consider all factors. That's why it's important for you to review all the fatigue stressors that might be fueling your fatigue so you can remove them from the equation.

In The Know

"Because major depression and chronic fatigue syndrome (CFS) have significant concurrence (26 percent), clinicians often find it difficult to differentiate between the disorders when evaluating."

—G. Tucker, Department of Psychiatry and Behavioral Sciences, University of Washington

Depression can be a symptom of CFS, so there are other factors to look at and consider before assuming you have a primary depressive disorder (meaning that depression is your main problem). It's also important to note that many people with CFS don't suffer from depression at all. But people with CFS can end up depressed for many reasons, including the enormous loss a person experiences because his life is so altered, the distress about the repercussions the illness is causing, the degree of physical suffering, and the frustration of not being able to actually do the activities he enjoys because he becomes sicker after activity.

Because CFS often leads to or contributes to very stressful socioeconomic situations, including poverty and social isolation, many people do become depressed. And it's a fact that some people with CFS spend so much time trying to convince others, including their doctors, that they have a real physical illness that they do become depressed. You can help your doctor figure out whether you have depression or CFS by knowing some facts that help differentiate the two. The following table outlines these.

Chronic Fatigue Syndrome	Depression
Overwhelming and debilitating postactivity fatigue and muscle weakness.	Constant feelings of being tired, typically associated with a lack of motivation or interest in all activities
Pain and fatigue due in part to inability to exercise	Pain and fatigue due in part to inactivity as a result of lack of desire
More flulike symptoms, headaches, abnormalities in deep-sleep brain wave patterns, more severe muscle and joint pain, Restless Legs Syndrome, and an increase in the incidence of colds and viruses	No extreme physical illness symptoms

continues

continued

Chronic Fatigue Syndrome	Depression
Remains highly motivated and takes pleasure in doing things she is capable of without sustained lowering of mood	Little to no interest in doing previously pleasurable activities
Distressed about not being physically able to engage in life	Little to no interest in engaging in life
Self-esteem remains intact, focus is on physical inabilities	Considerably lower self-esteem along with more thought distortions, including focusing on the negative and internalizing their situations
Focus is on physical symptoms, perceives medical causes as the source of her illness	Typically believes her depression stems from psychological factors

The problem is, though, that the longer your severe fatigue continues without CFS-like physical symptoms, such as a sore throat, aches and pains, or fever, the more likely your diagnosis will be depression. You can have depression along with CFS or any other medical condition. Unfortunately, depression and fatigue reinforce each other in a vicious cycle. By considering, addressing, and taking every variable out of the equation—including depression and other fatigue stressors in your life—you will have a better chance of recovering sooner from your fatigue. It's often said that depression is anger turned inward. If you are having a difficult time expressing anger, you should get some support so that you learn how it can be handled in healthy ways. Anger is not a bad thing; instead it's a healthy, normal reaction to frustration and feelings of disrespect. By learning how to express your feelings, you can prevent feelings of depression. By venting, receiving validation of your feelings, processing, and letting go of the situation (forgetting about it), you can get through times of frustration without becoming chronically angry or depressed.

Anxiety

A majority of people with fatigue syndromes also have anxiety, so it's thought that chronic fatigue is also a symptom or an expression of some anxiety disorders. Some common signs of anxiety are feeling on edge, tension, fatigue, lack of or low energy, worrying, self-doubt and indecisiveness, difficulty problem-solving, worry about social situations or performance, perfectionism, a tendency to procrastinate, addictive behaviors, depression, trouble controlling emotions or thoughts, and a tendency to be highly sensitive.

Anxiety can be triggered by stress, but some people are just more vulnerable to anxiety than others. And anxiety also can be a symptom related to other fatigue stressors such as a poor diet that leads to feelings of continual hypoglycemia or low blood sugar. Hypoglycemia has symptoms of anxiety—such as sweating, trembling, and feeling dizzy—so both of them reinforce each other. Anxiety also can be a result of negative self-talk or that inner voice that is always telling you the worst will happen.

> **Energy Bar** _____
>
> Important self-help methods to aid in the management of anxiety are stress-reduction techniques, dealing with excessive behavior problems (including addictions), a good diet and sleep habits, regular exercise, getting rid of toxic people and relationships, and learning to love and care for yourself.

Anger and Rage

Anger can be caused or worsened by frustration, feeling disrespected, physical or mental exhaustion or fatigue, pain, alcohol and drugs, stress, and other irritations. Both anger and rage affect your body in the same way as stimulants do, jacking up the stress response. You need to realize and be aware that less-obvious but equally damaging stimulants are arguing, hatred, loud music, movies and news that have frightening or suspenseful contents, sexual preoccupations, and addictions and other thrill-seeking behavior.

Many people use stimulants to give them temporary energy because they are stressed and approaching burnout. Angry, nervous people who have difficulty controlling their moods have a constant, internal, damaging stress response going on. This sort of wear and tear eventually leads to fatigue related to adrenal burnout. Continual pressure flogs your adrenal glands and they will, after a time, just give out.

If you experience fatigue due to adrenal burnout, you will be even less able to deal with irritation and frustration. So if you've been driving in the fast lane for too long, you might have a tendency to use the stress hormones generated by behaviors like road rage to function. Anger, rage, other stimulants, and fatigue then fuel each other in a vicious circle. When you find yourself chronically angry … ding, ding, ding … that's a clue you need some balance, with healthy time-outs for some real rest and relaxation. And when the content, magnitude, and frequency of your anger doesn't fit the situations, you might have what they call displaced anger and anger management classes might be in order.

Eating Disorders

Even though they might not appear to be very thin or very overweight, a lot of people suffer with *eating disorders*. Men and women with these disorders have all different body weights ranging from very thin and wasted to morbidly obese. People with compulsive eating disorder can be underweight, and those with anorexia nervosa can be slightly overweight. So someone's appearance does not necessarily indicate the severity of her disease, which is why many people suffer in silence while their families and others don't have a clue how sick they are.

def•i•ni•tion

Eating disorders include anorexia nervosa, a refusal to eat sufficient food to maintain a minimally normal body weight sometimes accompanied by obsessive exercise; bulimia nervosa, which includes episodes of binge eating, followed by ways of trying to purge the food from the body including self-induced vomiting, laxatives, and diuretics; and binge-eating disorder, the frequent episodes of uncontrollable overeating of abnormally large amounts without purging.

Poor and imbalanced eating habits and behaviors such as starvation, laxative use, and purging take their toll on the body. They result in electrolyte imbalances, vitamin and mineral deficiencies, depression, malnutrition, weakness, fatigue, heart problems, muscle wasting, and even death.

In today's society, due to media and other pressures, there is an unhealthy emphasis on physical appearance—most notably on the importance of thinness for any type of success. But the development of eating disorders goes beyond a desire to be thin; it is an indication and manifestation of low self-esteem, distorted self-image, and poor coping mechanisms. An eating-disordered person uses her distorted eating behaviors to give her a better sense of control. These behaviors allow for a temporary escape from feelings of depression, anxiety, stress, anger, and guilt. These ill people typically have unrealistically high expectations of themselves that continually cause them to fall short and suffer feelings of low self-esteem.

The tendency to overvalue physical appearance in their self-evaluation is out of balance, and all their self-worth is tied to appearance rather than other accomplishments such as school or career achievement. If a person with an eating disorder, for example, achieves a major success in school or work, it will be completely disregarded by that individual if she has not met her current weight, exercise, or eating goals.

Eating disorders have a profound impact on a person's quality of life and long-term health. Behaviors like starvation, purging, compulsive exercise, and binging can radically alter normal physiology. This can cause and lead to crippling health problems such as devastating conditions like CFS and even death. Like other disorders, these do not typically exist in a vacuum and people ill with eating disorders often have other mitigating problems. Getting help is of utmost importance to nip the potential for other real and damaging problems down the line.

Toxic Relationships

You don't have to ingest or inhale toxins to be poisoned; you can suffer the same adverse health effects from toxic relationships including chronic fatigue, insomnia, and many other ailments. Toxic people aren't just those who are negative, angry, or difficult—they can be cunningly manipulative, playing mind games with you that cause your insides to turn and your emotions to plummet. Because many toxic people might not show that poisonous side to anyone but you, they can cause an extra internal battle of the continual, "Is it me?"

These sorts of people typically require a sort of unilateral relationship because it's all about them. They set the pace, they make the rules, and they say what is okay for you to say or do and what is not. They aren't really interested in you; therefore, anything that has to do with you takes the spotlight off of them and causes them to react with criticism, unsolicited advice, hostility, silence, or irritation. There might not be a give-and-take because your issues are a burden to them, and they will let you know! In other words, toxic relationships won't support your healing and move toward positive changes because they are countersupportive.

If you find yourself involved with someone who you feel you can't be yourself around, that's also a sign of a toxic person or relationship. Toxic people are very often perfectionists who require perfection in others as much as themselves. While you don't hear their internal dialogue, what you do hear continually is what they don't like about you—and at inappropriate times and in inappropriate places.

Don't be swayed by your conscience because toxic people are masters of the guilt trip; they first upset you, then set you up, and then blame you for any outcomes. Although volumes have been written about how to identify toxic people, it always comes down to how another person makes you feel. If someone is making you feel bad, that person is toxic in your life.

You can have a toxic relationship with anyone: friends, parents, brothers, sisters, boyfriends and girlfriends, work colleges, and spouses. The feelings of anger, upset, misunderstanding, and betrayal they cause you to have can also lead to fatigue, exhaustion, and even such serious problems as heart attacks.

Getting rid of these toxic relationships sometimes can be complicated, particularly if family, money, jobs, or other certain extenuating circumstances exist. You first need to understand that you matter and that you have to put out the effort to either confront the person, limit the time you spend with him, or sever the relationship completely. For the purposes of healing, it's of utmost importance to, at the very least, understand that "It's not you!"

Grief

Grief is the normal expected response to a loss or a major life-changing event including an intense disappointment. Every individual experiences grief in her own way, but there are five definite stages in the grief process: denial and isolation, anger, bargaining, depression, and acceptance.

Grief commonly has physical manifestations that include fatigue, insomnia, anorexia, tightness in the chest, shortness of breath, feelings of choking, menstrual irregularities, and gastrointestinal disturbances. Bereaved people tend to eat less and sleep poorly as they experience life-altering changes and conflicting emotions. The feelings of anger, loneliness, sadness, shame, anxiety, and guilt can lead to physical and mental illness.

The work of grief has three distinct tasks for a mourner, including dealing with the initial shock and adjustment, a reconstruction of belief systems and acceptance, and reclaiming and going on with life. Those who get the support they need can work through the stages with fewer demands on the mind and body. Adjusting to life after the grieving process involves this important work, but all the tasks require considerable effort that can lead to overwhelming fatigue.

The average bereavement period can typically last up to one year. If you are finding that you are not able to get over a traumatic life event, especially one that may have occurred years ago, seek the help of a professional to help you work through your grief.

Substance Abuse Withdrawal

There are many symptoms of substance abuse, but they certainly include very poor mental and physical health and sometimes extreme fatigue. The person using drugs also might experience personality changes; social withdrawal; or a decreased interest in work, school, and relationships.

Substance-related disorders include the use of alcohol, amphetamines, inhalants, morphine, heroin, marijuana, cocaine, hallucinogens, methamphetamine, and PCP. These substances typically cause some sort of intoxication, along with a level of dependence, abuse, and subsequent withdrawal.

Because addictive behaviors are associated with fatigue, you need to recognize whether they are a problem for you. Hallmark traits include obsession, seeking out and engaging in the behavior, using despite knowing the negative consequences, compulsive behavior, withdrawal symptoms, loss of control, denial, concealing the behavior, episodic blackouts, depression, and low self-esteem.

The withdrawal symptoms vary with the substance being used, but some of the symptoms include fatigue (sometimes extreme), increased heart rate, trembling, insomnia, and irritability. People with substance abuse problems typically have multiple issues that are stressing their minds and bodies so they often need comprehensive treatment.

Slip-Ups

Caffeine, nicotine, compulsive gambling, and sexual addictions also fall into the rubric of substance abuse. Be aware of these addictive behaviors because they also can carry some of the health risks and consequences that using illegal substances and abusing prescription medications do.

Medication Withdrawal

Although doctors prescribe medications, the drug addiction you can experience from prescription medications has the same real and devastating consequences of any substance you can get off the street. Many people are lured into a false sense of safety and even legitimacy with prescription drug use and often are naive about the potential for addiction. For the record, prescription drug addiction is as powerful as that of heroin addiction with an equally grueling detox. And, just because you are getting your drugs from a doctor, it doesn't reduce your risk for addiction. With long-term use beyond what is recommended for certain drugs, a person typically first develops a *tolerance* for the drug, then becomes *dependant*, and sadly some become *addicted* to prescription drugs. Some of the most commonly abused drugs are the following:

◆ Opioids that are used to treat pain, including morphine, codeine, oxycodone, Vicodin (hydrocodone), and Demerol (meperedine).

◆ Central nervous system depressants used to treat anxiety, panic attacks, and sleep disorders, including Nembutal (pentobarbital sodium) and benzodiazepines such as Valium (diazepam) and Xanax (alprazolam).

◆ Central nervous system stimulants used to treat the sleep disorder narcolepsy and attention-deficit hyperactivity disorder (ADHD), including Ritalin (methylphenidate) and Dexedrine (dextroamphetamine).

def•i•ni•tion

Tolerance is a decrease in the effects of a drug with continual use. Physical **dependence** is characterized by the development of withdrawal symptoms and/or behavior changes when the drug is stopped or the dose is abruptly reduced. **Addiction** causes dysfunctional behavior including denial of drug use, lying, stealing drugs from friends or family members, forging prescriptions, selling and buying drugs on the street, and using prescribed drugs to get stoned or high.

Depending on the drug, withdrawal symptoms can vary but may include fatigue (sometimes extreme), depression, and disturbance of sleep patterns.

Antidepressants also can cause a withdrawal reaction, sometimes called *antidepressant discontinuation reaction* or *SSRI discontinuation syndrome*. Although the incidence and prevalence of this withdrawal syndrome isn't known, it is known that the severity of the symptoms can range from minor to severe. The symptoms can include dizziness, vertigo, light-headedness, nausea and vomiting, fatigue, headache, insomnia, and other sometimes frightening and uncomfortable symptoms such as shocklike sensations.

Withdrawal symptoms caused by prescription drug addiction all depend on various factors. You need to always consider the type of drug, the dose, the potency of the drug, the duration of action and length of using the drug, the reason it was prescribed, individual personalities and lifestyles, other stressors and past experiences, and the degree of support you have available. Many people require professional help and support to withdraw or discontinue prescription medications. You certainly need to be monitored by your doctor when you discontinue use of any potentially addictive drug or a drug that can cause withdrawal symptoms.

The Least You Need to Know

- ◆ Fatigue is a major symptom of many psychiatric disorders, so it's likely your doctor will consider a psychological cause if you check out medically.

- ◆ Continual stress makes you even more vulnerable to everyday pressures, including mental health problems such as anxiety and depression, while it weakens your immune system function and sets you up for becoming burned out or getting sick.

- ◆ A majority of people with fatigue syndromes also have anxiety, so it's thought that chronic fatigue is a symptom or expression of some anxiety disorders.

- ◆ You can suffer the same adverse health effects as poisons from toxic relationships, anger, rage, stimulants, and substance abuse, including chronic fatigue, insomnia, and many other ailments.

- ◆ Grief commonly has physical manifestations that include fatigue, insomnia, anorexia, tightness in the chest, shortness of breath, feelings of choking, menstrual irregularities, and gastrointestinal disturbances.

Part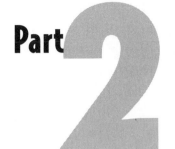

Taking Charge of Your Fatigue

Most of the time fatigue is not due to a medical condition, but you still need to get checked out by your doctor. Regardless of whether you have a medical problem, you still can take advantage of medicine and alternative methods such as acupuncture, supplements, and massage. This part covers how conventional medicine and alternative treatments and methods can help treat some causes, alleviate symptoms, and even positively impact the mind-body system to abolish fatigue and achieve an improved quality of life.

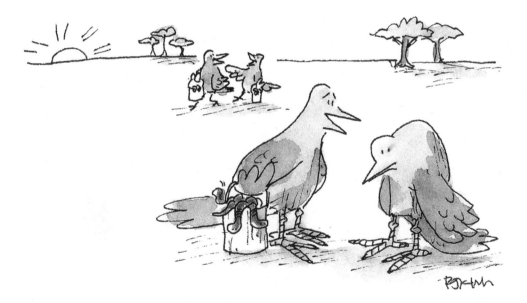

"Where ya' been, Jack? Unlike you—haven't made it in time once this week."

Chapter 6

How Your Doctor Can Help

In This Chapter

- ◆ Uncovering your diagnosis
- ◆ Working with your medical provider
- ◆ Basic and specialized medical tests
- ◆ Are you depressed?

So far, this book has focused on explaining and describing fatigue; understanding signs, symptoms, and signals; and identifying contributing factors. Hopefully you've been able to connect some of the dots to figure out what some of the causes of fatigue are.

Seeing your doctor is important to rule out any treatable medical or psychological causes of your fatigue. Knowing how to prepare for your doctor visit, what to expect, and how to partner with your doctor will give you the best advantage.

Your first appointment is an assessment and examination to give your doctor the necessary information to come up with a diagnosis or clues as where to go next. Even if your doctor suspects a psychological cause, chances are you will still have lab studies done to confirm that there is nothing medically wrong.

Getting Started

You can help your doctor by monitoring and documenting your fatigue in writing before you go in. You could use the Fatigue Severity Scale outlined in Chapter 9 or use a scale from one to ten to describe your level of fatigue. Document when your energy levels are highest and lowest and how fatigue impacts your day-to-day activities, including work and leisure.

Providing specifics regarding your symptoms and the impact they are having on your life is much more useful than simply saying fatigue is interfering with your life. For example, a hallmark of severe fatigue (like CFS) is the worsening of fatigue and other symptoms after physical or mental activity, known as post exertional malaise. By recording your symptoms, you might also uncover what makes your symptoms worse and what makes them better—all useful information to your doctor and helpful to you to identify your *fatigue triggers*.

Your social history, including alcohol use, drug use, smoking, and where you work are all important information. The first three are obvious; the last might bring up clues to any toxic exposures or clues to sleep deprivation. Give your doctor personal information even if you are uncomfortable or embarrassed doing so because it might be needed for your diagnosis. Write all your questions down before you get there so you don't get overwhelmed and forget to ask certain burning questions. Remember, too, that you have limited time with your doctor so being prepared will give you the best advantage. If you don't understand something, be sure to ask your doctor to write it down. Also find out about after-hour staffing, who to call if you need additional help, or where to go for more information.

def•i•ni•tion

Your personal **fatigue triggers** can include stress, perfumes and fragrances, mold, certain foods, skipping meals, environmental temperatures, or excess caffeine or sugar in your diet.

Talking to Your Doctor

Most doctors have a medical history form for you to fill out, but if you want to be more thorough you can make up your own history ahead of time to bring to your appointment. Include all illnesses, diseases, conditions, hospitalizations and surgeries, dates, and reasons in the past and present.

Your family history can uncover links to help you get a diagnosis. Some of the more common markers for fatiguing illnesses are a personal or family history of irritable bowel syndrome, thyroid disease, mental illnesses, endometriosis, miscarriage, mononu-cleosis, autoimmune diseases, and chronic infections including ear and sinus infections.

Don't forget to mention any piercings or tattoos, blood transfusions, or history of IV drug use, no matter how long it has been since you got them. Some chronic infections have been traced back to both because, whenever you puncture the skin, you create a portal of entry for infectious organisms.

Let you doctor know about any viral illnesses you've had because there may be some connection to your chronic fatigue. And the fatiguing effects of any recent flu, colds, or infections might linger for weeks or months, also weakening your ability to deal with other stressors—particularly if you are not taking care of yourself in other areas of your life (mind-body imbalance).

List your current and past medications and be as accurate as you can be, including the name of the medication, the dose and frequency, and the reason for taking it. Don't forget to list any over-the-counter (OTC) medications, vitamins, supplements, and herbs you are taking. Many medications and combinations of medications, both pre-scription and OTC, can cause or contribute to fatigue.

Tell your doctor about any traumas and injuries, toxic exposures, extreme stress, per-fectionism, and type-A personality characteristics because these might be causing or contributing to your fatigue. Don't forget to mention other major stressors like post-traumatic stress disorder; or emotional, physical, or sexual abuse; and history of eating disorders.

Part of your medical history is giving your doctor clues to piece together a picture of what your fatigue looks like, acts like, and is affected by. Let your doctor know what was going on in your life when the fatigue started. By gauging how long you have been feeling fatigued, you might uncover possible links and causes such as stressors or a recent illness.

It's important to consider whether your fatigue is constant or if it comes and goes. Think about if you ever experienced the same symptoms, and what they were related to, such as an illness or a particular stressor. Report any diagnosis you had then and any treatment.

If you think sleep is a factor, let your doctor know how much sleep you get every night and if you do shift work or travel frequently. You might be sleep deprived or experiencing sleep disorder problems related to working off shifts. Other important information is a history of snoring, insomnia, and any other behaviors that might be interfering with your sleep.

Narrowing Your Diagnosis

Be honest about any substance abuse problems and addiction problems, even if you presently have no intentions of dealing with them. Tell your doctor about any symptoms of hypoglycemia, poor eating habits such as skipping meals or a low-nutrient diet, overuse of caffeine, headaches, night sweats, brain fog, thinking and memory problems, panic attacks and other mood problems, and dental or jaw problems.

Your doctor might ask you about other aspects of your life to better understand your history of fatigue, including any unusual events like a family member passing away, a stressful move, a job layoff, or increased job responsibilities. Other factors that are important for your doctor to consider in your diagnosis are the following:

◆ Do you practice safe sex or birth control? Fatigue is a symptom of HIV and hepatitis B that might be acquired through sexual activity. Pregnancy often results in fatigue.

◆ Have you had any unexplained weight loss or gain? You might be hyper- or hypothyroid, diabetic, or anemic, or you may have depression or anxiety.

◆ Are you nervous, restless, or irritable? Do you feel bored, stressed, or disappointed? You might be experiencing burnout, anxiety, or other stress- and mood-related problems.

◆ Is your exhaustion constant and extreme, and does it follow minimal exertion? Do you also have headaches and brain fog, aching joints and muscle pain, sore throat, and swollen lymph glands? You might have CFS or fibromyalgia.

◆ Do you also have a husky voice, constipation, cold intolerance, and hair loss? You might be hypothyroid.

◆ Do you have frequent urination, excessive thirst, and weight loss? You might be diabetic.

◆ Do you have heart palpitations, hot flashes, and night sweats? You might be perimenopausal.

Slip-Ups

Eyestrain related to sustained use of a computer can also cause fatigue. Relieve eyestrain by using ergonomically correct workstation conditions, practicing good posture, wearing computer glasses, using special antiglare screens, and doing eye exercises.

And finally mention any fever, breathlessness when lying down, impotence or a change in sex drive, bronze discoloration of the skin, muscle weakness, nausea and diarrhea, intolerance to heat, increased sweating, restless sleep, and morning headaches. These are all symptoms of conditions that might be causing your fatigue.

It's Your Doctor's Turn

Your doctor will begin by doing a problem-directed history and physical that might provide enough information to result in a diagnosis. Your physical exam should include a skin check; a head, eyes, ears, nose, and throat exam; and a pulse, weight, and blood pressure check. Your doctor will examine your neck to look at your thyroid, listen to your heart and lungs, feel the organs in your abdomen, and do a brief neurological exam.

A primary care physician, a family doctor, an internist, or a general practitioner will be able to diagnose the most common conditions that cause fatigue. But the best doctor to assess, evaluate, and treat your fatigue will be one who is able to appreciate that fatigue is a problem for you, take the time to listen to your concerns, understand enough about fatigue to do a proper evaluation, and be willing to go the distance with you even if that means referring you to another doctor or specialist.

Fatigue, tiredness, sleepiness, and lack of energy are some of the most common complaints doctors hear, and it sometimes takes some investigative work for them to understand and diagnose. Your doctor needs to figure out if your problem is sleep deprivation or chronic fatigue that is associated with a certain condition, a mind-body imbalance, or a combination of causes.

In The Know

"People with CFS have reduced overall cortisol output within the first hour after they wake up in the morning, which is actually one of the most stressful times for the body. We need further studies to better understand the relationship between morning cortisol levels and functional status of a patient suffering from CFS."

—William C. Reeves, M.D., Centers for Disease Control and Prevention

---

How to Get the Best Care

Bring something to write with so you can take notes. Some people even like to tape record their visits, but be sure to ask first if it's alright to do so. It's even okay to bring a friend or family member with you, especially if that person has been badgering you about some symptom or behavior, you get nervous around doctors, or you are very ill.

If you see other doctors, keep all of them informed on your various treatments and tests. Call for any test results and ask what the test results mean. Also, be sure to schedule follow-up appointments, let your doctor know how the treatment is working, and make appointments with any specialists your doctor wants you to see.

Ask questions and be sure you understand the answers. The following is information you might find out at this visit or subsequent visits:

- What your diagnosis is

- The cause(s) of your condition

- The recommended treatment or lifestyle changes

- The risks and benefits of the treatments

- Any prescribed medication, including its side effects, how long it takes to feel the effects, and exactly how to take it

- The measures you can take

- What your prognosis is

Necessary Tests

Lab tests help your doctor exclude some of the minor and some of the more treatable causes of fatigue. Even if your doctor doesn't feel your fatigue is a medically treatable problem, you should still have labs done if only to give you the proof that there is nothing there so you can focus on other causative factors. Your doctor will send you to a lab to have some routine blood tests that might include a complete blood count (CBC), an erythrocyte sedimentation rate (sed rate), thyroid tests, a chemistry or metabolic panel including electrolytes and glucose level, and a urinalysis (UA).

Laboratory Tests

Some basic laboratory tests can be useful in ruling out possible physical causes for your fatigue. Depending on your history and physical, your risks, recent travels, or exposures, you might also get some other tests. To rule out the more common causes, your doctor may perform the following tests:

- A CBC (or just one part of that test such as hemoglobin, hematocrit, or white blood cell count) checks you for infections, anemia, allergic and toxic reactions, and many other disorders.

◆ Erythrocyte Sedimentation Rate, or Sed rate, is a test for inflammation in your body due to such inflammatory conditions as thyroid disease, rheumatoid arthritis, and lupus.

◆ *Thyroid-stimulating hormone (TSH)* rules out a thyroid condition.

def•i•ni•tion

According to the American Association of Clinical Endocrinologists, the **normal thyroid-stimulating hormone (TSH)** range is 0.3 to 3.0. Previously, a TSH above 5.5 would have been considered hypothyroid, but the newer guidelines indicate that a TSH above 3.0 might be diagnosed as hypothyroid.

◆ Tuberculosis screening (PPD skin test).

◆ Carboxyhemoglobin is a test that rules out carbon-monoxide poisoning.

◆ Antibody test to rule out hepatitis B or C.

◆ Ferritin rules out iron deficiency.

◆ Urinalysis screens for many illnesses and conditions.

◆ Urine toxicology screen shows any toxins you might be exposed to or levels of drugs you might be taking.

◆ A chemistry (metabolic) panel measures the levels of certain chemical substances from various tissues in your body.

You might get a portion of the chemistry panel or a more complete or comprehensive metabolic panel including the following:

◆ Electrolytes (sodium, potassium, calcium, chloride, and carbon dioxide) are tested because they are crucial for body system balance and function and abnormal components indicate a wide range of clinical problems and conditions. Blood glucose level checks for possible diabetes.

◆ Albumin tests for a number of conditions, including primary liver disease, tissue damage or inflammation, malabsorption syndromes, malnutrition, and kidney diseases.

◆ Globulin levels are checked for cirrhosis of the liver.

◆ Blood urea nitrogen (BUN) and creatinine level test check your kidney function for presence of dehydration. Albumin checks out your liver and kidneys. The bilirubin test checks liver function and signs of liver disease, such as hepatitis or cirrhosis, or the effects of medicines on the liver. It also indicates obstructions of the bile ducts such as gallstones or tumors of the pancreas and suggests conditions that cause an increased destruction of red blood cells.

◆ Alkaline phosphatase (ALP) checks for liver disease, damage to the liver, bone problems, or the cause of a high blood calcium level. The aspartate aminotransferase (AST) test looks for causes of liver damage, helps to diagnose liver disease (especially hepatitis and cirrhosis), and monitors recovery from or treatment for liver disease. The alanine aminotransferase (ALT) test helps to diagnose liver disease—particularly cirrhosis and hepatitis caused by alcohol, drugs, or viruses such as hepatitis B and C—and checks for liver damage.

Specialized Diagnostic Tests

Depending on your symptoms, your history, and the results of your initial tests, you might then also have additional specialized tests including the following. However, some of these tests might also have been done with your first set of labs.

◆ A test for Lyme disease

◆ Labs to check for autoimmune disease including ANA, Rheumatoid factor to test for rheumatoid arthritis, and tests for lupus

◆ A VDRL and rapid plasma reagin test to screen for syphilis

◆ HIV test (requires a signed consent from you to perform)

◆ Blood tests to check you for any muscle disease

◆ Cortisol level for adrenal problems

◆ Antithyroid antibodies if you have a TSH abnormality in the first test

◆ Blood cultures to test you for infection if you have a long-standing fever

◆ X-rays, a bone scan, an upper GI series, and tests to examine your small bowel and kidney function

◆ Muscle biopsy to test for certain collagen and muscle diseases

Some people have an elevated TSH level without having the other lab findings that are necessary to diagnose hypothyroidism. They also suffer from symptoms of hypothyroid such as dry skin, cold intolerance, and easy fatigability. This is where it gets tricky because some doctors treat this subclinical hypothyroid state but some choose to wait until the lab studies are more definitive.

If you have fatigue, dry skin, cold intolerance, constipation, muscle cramps, or other common symptoms of hypothyroidism but your lab studies don't support the diagnosis, it might be best to see an endocrinologist. There is a lot going on, including continual changes in the way this condition is being diagnosed and treated, and a specialist will be on top of any current changes.

The test for hypoglycemia is a five-hour glucose tolerance test in which you drink a sugar solution and blood is drawn at various intervals and tested. Many people have normal blood sugar values on this test even with symptoms of hypoglycemia.

For any symptoms or suspicions of neurological disease such as multiple sclerosis, you will also be referred to a neurologist for further testing such as an imaging test called magnetic resonance imaging (MRI). If there is any possibility that you might have sleep apnea, you might also undergo an overnight test in a sleep clinic. Depending on the results of your blood tests, you might need additional workups that your doctor will discuss with you.

In The Know

It was once believed that immunologic tests had a place in diagnosing fatiguing illness. But today according to the CDC, immunologic tests such as measurements of natural killer cell (NK), cytokine tests (interleukin-1, interleukin-6, or interferon), or cell marker tests (CD25 or CD16) have no value for diagnosing CFS.

Checking your stool for blood is a way to determine anemia caused by bleeding in your stomach or intestines. Your doctor might check that in the office after a rectal exam or give you a kit for you to get the sample at home and bring back to the office or lab. More tests are necessary if blood is found in the stool, such as an endoscopy in which a tube with a very small camera is used to view the lining of the digestive tract. Bone marrow aspiration and biopsy tests might be done to check whether your bone marrow is unhealthy and whether you are making enough blood cells. If you need any of these additional tests, you will be well-prepared by your doctor beforehand.

Assessing Depression

The majority of doctors consider depression as a diagnosis if your routine lab tests are normal even though there aren't any blood tests or x-rays that can tell you if you are depressed. Sometimes you might have fatigue for reasons other than depression, but you become depressed as a result of how the fatigue is impacting your life. It's important to look at any signs of major depression so you can address it as a separate issue. The standard questions to evaluate depression include the following:

During the last two weeks at least …

♦ Have you felt sad or down in the dumps the majority of the time and more often than you have felt in the past?

♦ Have you felt tired with no energy?

♦ Do you find it difficult to concentrate?

♦ Have you had trouble with sleeping too much or not being able to sleep?

♦ Have you been eating too much or too little?

♦ Have you been crying for no reason?

♦ Have you had difficulty enjoying activities you normally enjoy?

♦ Have you felt guilty for no reason?

♦ Have you felt that things are going to go wrong and are out of your control?

Energy Bar _____

Exercise or engage in some sort of physical activity to help protect you against depression because physical deconditioning often increases or even causes fatigue.

The Importance of Correct Diagnosis

Your fatigue might be a symptom of one or more treatable conditions, or it might be a result of an overall mind-body imbalance you need to identify and take steps to correct. Don't be afraid to find out what's wrong because many causes of fatigue are treatable and many are completely fixable.

If your doctor is not finding any diagnosis but you are absolutely certain that something is wrong, get a second opinion. Some doctors are better than others at working with less well-defined subjective symptoms and conditions. You might have a condition that your doctor is not that familiar with or has not yet tested you for. There are no lab tests, imaging studies, or scans to diagnose fibromyalgia, CFS, and depression, but all these are conditions that can be treated with various medications, therapies, and lifestyle changes.

You might have a sleep disorder such as insomnia that is independent of depression, or you might have hepatitis B or C regardless of whether you feel you had prior risk factors for infection. Work with your doctor so you can narrow down any possible causes, get the maximum benefit from the available treatment options, and then maximize the benefits even further by doing your part. You probably don't understand how much of your life has been affected by your fatigue until long after the smoke clears and you begin to feel much better.

Even though you might be at a place where you are desperate to know that something is wrong so it can be fixed, no news is still good news. It's much better to have something fixable in your lifestyle than to have a medical diagnosis you have to live with the rest of your life.

The Least You Need to Know

- A complete medical and social history and a physical exam are necessary to rule out any medical conditions.

- Keeping track of your symptoms and what makes them better or worse and documenting how your symptoms are affecting your life will help your doctor to find the correct diagnosis and help you identify any triggers.

- Basic laboratory tests are part of a workup to discover the cause of your fatigue.

- You might have additional tests done in subsequent visits to help narrow down your diagnosis.

- There aren't any lab tests to diagnose depression, but you will be evaluated by answering some basic questions.

Chapter 7

Medical Options

In This Chapter

◆ A look at prescription and over-the-counter medications

◆ Off-label uses for symptom relief

◆ How to use drugs intelligently and judiciously

◆ Treating certain conditions can improve fatigue

◆ Why body work can help improve fatigue

While your focus in winning your fight needs to be primarily on correcting lifestyle issues such as poor eating and sleeping habits, creating balance, reducing stress, and eliminating toxins, you may also need to treat some of your symptoms and problems with medication. Remember that only 10 percent of fatigued people have an underlying medical condition. Therefore, fatigue is largely a lifestyle problem, so most people just need a little help with issues such as pain and insomnia to get the restorative rest needed to get back on track.

Because nothing exists in a vacuum and your fatigue has far-reaching effects, the collateral damage can be anxiety, depression, or it can worsen problems such as insomnia. Keep in mind that this book is about treating fatigue and not about treating major depression, so recommendations here are for treating fatigue fallout so to speak. This is not a comprehensive source for treating a condition that has fatigue as a symptom. If you are depressed, you should see a doctor.

There is no single recommended prescription treatment for chronic fatigue. There are, however, medications you can use to help with certain symptoms, medical conditions, and/or aggravating illnesses that you have along with your fatigue. Talk to your doctor in order to find out your best options based on your own personal health history and present concerns.

Prescription Medications

The best way to look at prescription medications is that they may be something to get you over the hump, even if that hump is the size of a mountain. Consider that you should target allergies for example with such things as an elimination diet and avoidance of allergens, sinus irrigation, and removal of toxic agents so that you can begin to restore a healthy immune system. Some people with Chronic Fatigue Syndrome (CFS), find they are unusually sensitive to certain medications, particularly those that act on the *central nervous system* (CNS). This is why you need to let your doctor know if you are experiencing adverse side effects and perhaps start with low doses and increase them only as necessary.

def•i•ni•tion

The **central nervous system (CNS)** consists of the brain and spinal column. It's possible that dysfunction of the CNS, the immune system, and the adrenal glands may be behind disorders like CFS and Fibromyalgia (FM).

While some think that medications interfere with certain vital sleep stages, the truth is that if you are not sleeping at all for any reason, or you are getting poor or interrupted sleep, or pain is preventing you from sleeping and doing any other healing work, then you need to get help from medications. Low doses of certain medications may help you get the restorative sleep that you need in order to heal. If you use medication as a bridge to get to the other side while working on other areas, the medication can be a helpful tool.

Antidepressants

According to CFS experts the use of antidepressants is helpful to alleviate pain, and to improve sleep, energy levels, and cognitive impairment in this devastating fatigue illness. If you have CFS *and* depression you might want to try one of the selective serotonin reuptake inhibitors (SSRI) or tricyclic antidepressants.

CFS experts have found that people who have true CFS tend to be overly sensitive to the effects of SSRIs when used for reasons other than depression. So it's worth discussing this with your doctor who might recommend using a lower dose or one half to one third of the usual dose if you have CFS. Talk to your doctor about what SSRI will be your best choice to improve symptoms such as pain, fatigue, and poor sleep.

Some of the older agents on the market are the tricyclic antidepressants such as amitriptyline, which, in small doses, may be helpful to promote sleep, decrease fibromyalgia pain, and help improve low energy levels. Like all antidepressants, the effects may not be apparent for up to three to four weeks, and you need to take the drug all the time, not just when you have pain. Report all side effects to your doctor.

Monoamine Oxidase Inhibitors (MAOIs) block the activity of a protein "monoamine oxidase" to prevent the breakdown of your brain's monoamine neurotransmitters (serotonin, norepinephrine, and dopamine) and to increase your available stores of neurotransmitters. Making neurotransmitters more available may help alleviate depressive symptoms associated with low stores of monoamine neurotransmitters. MAOIs may also be helpful in restoring energy levels in people with fatigue but who also carry a risk of severe hypertension caused by eating certain foods that have a high tyramine content. These foods include aged cheeses, most red wines, sauerkraut, vermouth, chicken livers, dried meats and fish, canned figs, fava beans, and concentrated yeast products. Because so many other options are available and MOAIs are risky, most doctors will choose other agents if possible.

The typical side effects of many antidepressants include dry eyes and mouth, and blurred vision. Side effects of tricyclics may also cause restlessness and decreased sexual drive. SSRI side effects may also include increased heart rate and constipation. Stopping these agents abruptly after using them for six weeks or more can cause a discontinuation syndrome, which includes symptoms of insomnia, anxiety, palpitations, headaches, and recurrent depression. To stop taking antidepressants, you may need to taper off them slowly over some time. Be sure to consult your doctor when it's time to stop these medications.

When you take any medication that causes dry mouth and eyes, and/or constipation, stay well hydrated and take omega-3 supplements in order to help stay regular and prevent other problems, such as tooth decay caused by decreased saliva.

Antianxiety

Antianxiety medications such as benzodiazepines and azapirones are mild tranquilizers that are commonly used to treat the symptoms of anxiety and panic. They can be useful for extreme pain that keeps you up at night, restless legs syndrome, and insomnia when used judiciously and intelligently. Some medications used for the treatment of depression have been also been found to relieve symptoms of anxiety including certain SSRIs, tricyclic antidepressants, MAOIs, and the newer atypical antidepressants such as duloxetine, mirtazapine, trazodone, and venlafaxine. Trazodone is a sedating antidepressant that may be also used in a low dose (50-250 milligrams) for anxiety related to fatigue. Risperidone is an antipsychotic drug that in low doses of up to one half milligram can help with pain, anxiety, and sleep.

Beta-blocker drugs are used to treat high blood pressure and heart problems and are also prescribed off-label for the treatment of anxiety. They work by blocking the effects of norepinephrine in order to alleviate the physiological symptoms of anxiety, including heart palpitations, sweating, tremors, and dizziness. Beta-blockers may help in anxiety-provoking situations such as stage fright, but they don't affect anxiety symptoms caused by emotional states such as worrying. Because one of the more common side effects of beta-blockers is fatigue, it might not be the best agent for you to use. Let your doctor know if you have any concerns.

In The Know

"Good nutrition is the foundation of natural treatment for anxiety. If you are serotonin-deficient you will crave sugar and simple carbohydrates. But those foods cause your insulin levels to spike and crash, further destabilizing your mood and creating that "bottoming out" feeling. Eat real whole foods, organic when possible, that will help maintain stable blood sugar levels. Avoid all processed, artificial products, trans fats, artificial additives, simple sugars and carbohydrates (or "white" food). Add multiple servings of fiber-rich vegetables or fruit to every meal and drink plenty of filtered water."

—Marcelle Pick, OB/GYN Nurse Practitioner—Women to Women's Healthcare Center, Yarmouth, Maine

---

Clonazepam is a benzodiazepine that can be used for sleep, pain, and anxiety in very small doses (one half milligram) and has been shown to actually decrease brain fog in some people with pain as their primary symptom.

According to the National Institute of Mental Health, benzodiazepines are addictive with prolonged use and it can take only a few weeks of regular use (everyday) to develop a tolerance to these drugs. You then need to up the dose to get the same effect, leading to dependence and addiction. That is why the National Institute of Mental Health recommends that these medications are prescribed for only brief periods, days or weeks, or just during stressful situations or anxiety attacks. It does acknowledge that some patients, however, do need long-term treatment. Any of the following are major signs that you may have a problem:

- ◆ Taking benzodiazepines for four months or longer.

- ◆ Relying on pills to cope.

- ◆ Feeling ill, anxious, or other unusual symptoms when not taking the pills.

- ◆ If you abruptly stop taking the drug, you experience severe withdrawal symptoms including agitation, insomnia, and rebound anxiety.

- ◆ A reduced effect occurs.

- ◆ You take a higher dose than prescribed for use "as needed" during times of stress or you exceed the dose that was prescribed for you to take on a regular basis.

- ◆ Cutting down or stopping your pills causes insomnia.

- ◆ You are drinking more or taking other drugs.

- ◆ You are sure that you always have a supply and always take the pills with you.

Pain

Tricyclic antidepressants (doxepin, amitriptyline, desipramine, and nortriptyline) in low doses might help improve sleep and relieve mild pain in CFS and FM. Some side effects of these medications are dry mouth, drowsiness, weight gain, and an elevated heart rate. Because some of the tricylcic drugs also reduce deep sleep, they may not be your best choice if you have insomnia.

Slip-Ups

Don't wait until your pain is severe before taking OTC or prescribed pain medication, because your medication works better and pain is easier to control when you first experience any symptoms and before it becomes full-blown. If you have chronic pain, you should probably take your pain medication on a regular basis or take it when you experience the beginning of pain.

Other medications that can be useful for pain are the following:

◆ Clonazepam (benzodiazepine) and venlafaxine (antidepressant) may also help increase your pain threshold so that you feel less pain.

◆ Some anticonvulsants such as gabapentin are also prescribed off-label for pain, Restless Legs Syndrome, and FDA approved for post herpetic neuralgia, which is a pain syndrome.

◆ Narcotic analgesics, although they carry a risk of addiction, are used for severe pain and to ease correlating joint and muscle stiffness related to fatigue.

◆ Muscle relaxants can be used to minimize muscle pain and muscle spasms.

◆ Tramadol can work well for treating insomnia and depression, but use it with caution in conjunction with certain SSRIs and tricyclics. It is a weak opiate related to the anti-inflammatory medications that don't contain cortisone called nonsteroidal anti-inflammatory drugs (NSAIDs [pronounced en-saydz]) and has some effect on the serotonin and norepinephrine systems.

Synthetic cortisone (a synthesized type of steroids or hormones produced by your adrenal gland) can be injected into a particular area of inflammation for a powerful anti-inflammatory effect to decrease pain. Cortisone injections are typically used to treat serious localized pain such as shoulder bursitis, arthritis, tennis elbow, and carpal tunnel syndrome.

NSAIDs are used to treat a wide variety of pain conditions that have a basis in inflammation, such as arthritis, bursitis, and tendonitis.

Allergy Drugs

Allergy medications don't cure allergies; however, they can help treat the symptoms that may cause or aggravate your fatigue. There is not a one-size-fits-all approach for allergy medication treatment; finding the right medication often takes trial and error. There are five major kinds of allergy medications: oral antihistamines, nasal antihistamines, decongestants, nasal sprays, and eye drops.

◆ Oral antihistamines work by blocking histamine, the chemical released by your body's immune system to help relieve sneezing, itching, nasal drainage, and hives. The most common side effect is drowsiness, which is why some antihistamines are also useful for insomnia and why you need to take care while using them and driving. It's also noteworthy that antihistamines may also inadvertently cause or aggravate your fatigue.

◆ Nasal antihistamines are sprayed directly into the nose where it is needed most.

◆ Decongestants are stimulants that work to reduce fluid buildup that blocks sinuses so they can by used for congestion caused by both colds and allergies. They are used to treat runny noses, swollen sinuses, and postnasal drip in various forms including pills, liquid, sprays, and drops. They don't, however, treat sneezing, itching, and nasal secretions. Decongestants can also cause insomnia, nervousness, difficulty with urination, headaches, and elevated blood pressure. They can cause a "rebound effect" when used for more than two or three consecutive days, causing your nasal congestion to become worse than it was before you started using it.

◆ Nonsteroid nasal sprays interfere with the release of histamine and are used to prevent allergy symptoms. Steroid type nasal sprays decrease inflammation and can counteract a greater variety of symptoms, such as congestion, postnasal drip, itching, and sneezing. Steroid nasal sprays decrease inflammation by opening the nasal passages; breathing through the nose is made easier.

Energy Bar

If you feel blah and desperate with chronic fatigue you just might have a sinus infection. Getting diagnosed can help you get rid of your fatigue.

◆ Eye drops are various medications that work to alleviate allergy symptoms that affect the eye or allergic conjunctivitis.

Hormonal Treatments

Thyroid hormone replacement is used to treat hypothyroidism. And while it's controversial, some believe that there is low thyroid activity in persons with conditions such as Chronic Fatigue Syndrome (CFS) and fibromyalgia. If you have symptoms of hypothyroidism with normal thyroid tests that are not detected by standard thyroid function tests (thyroid-stimulating hormone [TSH]), this condition is known as subclinical hypothyroidism. Some medical practitioners who are experts in endocrinology treat symptoms of hypothyroid with a normal TSH level when you have other validating factors, such as low tissue thyroid levels.

The most common thyroid replacements are Synthroid, Cytomel, Levoxyland, and Armour Thyroid. Some people feel that Armour Thyroid may have fewer side effects while giving them more balanced thyroid replacement and blood levels. Finding the right balance of thyroid hormone can be tricky, particularly if you have other compounding factors such as adrenal burnout caused by long-term intense stress. The recommendations for treatment of hypothyroidism is highly individual. As with all medical treatments, working with your doctor to find what works for you is the best bet.

The body's response to stress involves the limbic system, the hypothalamus, the pituitary gland, and the adrenal glands. These systems together are called the hypothalamic-pituitary-adrenal (HPA) axis. The cascade of events during stress is first the release of CRF (cortisol releasing factor) from the hypothalamus; this alerts the pituitary gland to secrete ACTH (adrenocorticotrophin hormone), signaling the adrenals to release cortisol into the bloodstream. After a period of chronic stress (burnout), the HPA axis can wear down and become dysfunctional. When the HPA axis system is dysfunctional, it can either fail to respond or fail to turn itself off after stress. CFS researchers like Jacob Teitelbaum, M.D., are beginning to think that CFS occurs due in part to the failed HPA axis response. Some doctors use low-dose cortisol (5 to 20 milligrams per day) in people with CFS and fibromyalgia to improve the HPA axis response with beneficial effects on symptoms.

Energy Bar

There's a lot of research happening in the antiaging department. Some reports indicate that aging is associated with changes in the dynamic function of the HPA axis and that these changes are weakened by aerobic fitness. So, cardio exercise is also good for hormone production and your mind-body balance!

In past years, the uncomfortable symptoms of menopause, including chronic fatigue, have been treated by doctors using synthetic hormone replacement. Because pharmaceutical companies are not able to patent a bioidentical compound, they invented synthetic hormones that have been widely used, but were found to be associated with serious adverse health effects including breast cancer, coronary heart disease, bone fractures, endometrial cancer, stroke, and blood clots.

The trend in treating menopausal changes and symptoms is the use of bioidentical hormone replacement that is made with the same molecular structure as the natural hormones in the body. Bioidentical hormones are metabolized in the same way as the natural body hormones, minimizing side effects. These more natural hormones are not a one-size-fits-all solution such as synthetic hormones are manufactured to be. Women should have their hormone levels checked with a simple blood test and replaced in a prescription such as Tri-Est and Bi-Est that are natural estrogen combination products that can be made at a compounding pharmacy to include progesterone. Both can be taken as pills or creams that are applied to the body. Hormone replacement is and has been a hot topic with constantly changing recommendations. As with any medical treatment, your best bet is to work with your doctor and follow a recommended treatment plan. Women and men alike should exercise, use stress-reduction techniques, eat a whole-food diet, and get the required sleep so that you can up your natural production of hormones!

Stimulants

Amantadine is an antiviral and an antiparkinsonic drug that also has a stimulant effect and reduces fatigue in some people with multiple sclerosis. Modafinil is a stimulant drug used to treat narcolepsy and shift work sleep disorder; it is marketed by the manufacturer for reducing excessive daytime sleepiness and improving alertness. Other stimulants such as dextroamphetamine and methylphenidate can be used to promote a sense of energy and well-being, but not without risk.

Choosing to use stimulants has to be weighed heavily against the obvious risk of dependence. Less obvious long-term risks are that you may overstimulate and further harm a potentially injured central nervous system and tired adrenal glands. So, consider when you use stimulants that they may make you feel well temporarily, but will eventually postpone your recovery or ultimately prevent it.

Vitamin B Injections

Dr. Paul Cheney, Dr. Jacob Teitelbaum, and Dr. Sarah Myhill are a few of the most highly respected CFS doctors and researchers who all recommend the use of vitamin B injections in patients with CFS. Although it's not an FDS approved treatment, they believe that there is some indication that intramuscular injections of vitamin B_{12} (3000 micrograms of cyanocobalamin) given twice per week might improve energy and well-being if you suffer fatigue. Although you can sense improvement within 12 to 24 hours of administration, because vitamin B is water-soluble and excreted in the urine, the effects tend to diminish after a few days, thus, the reason for repeat doses. It's thought that people with CFS might have abnormal B_{12} metabolism with an inability to transport B_{12} across the cell membrane and that supplementing may improve mood and cognitive ability while decreasing irritability, numbness, and weakness. If you consider B_{12} injections, you need to also be aware of the following:

◆ Your blood levels in lab tests might not reflect a deficiency, so you may consider B_{12} even if you have normal lab test results.

◆ You have to be okay with taking regular injections because oral or nasal spray preparations are not as effective as the injections.

◆ Results might take up to six weeks, so be patient.

◆ You can give yourself the shots at home after your doctor prescribes them and shows you how to do them.

◆ Tell your doctor immediately about any side effects including rash, skin discoloration, chills, or any other reaction following the shots.

◆ Make sure to take a quality multivitamin every day because B_{12} may affect the absorption of other vitamins.

◆ There isn't any worry about reaction with other medications or supplements.

Antimicrobials

Although many have looked and tried to find infections like Epstein Barr or Candida ablicans (yeast) as a source and cause of CFS, there just isn't any proof. The truth is that antibiotics, antivirals, or antifungal agents are not a proven or accepted treatment for CFS.

Some doctors do prescribe the antibiotic doxycycline in CFS for people with evidence of a recent infection (as shown by elevated blood IgM C pneumoniae titers). If you have an underlying infection, you need to take the treatment of choice for that infection.

In The Know
According to doctors the best approach to prevent infections like the flu is to boost your immune system, practice good hand washing and social distancing—staying away from sick people, especially during flu season. The CDC and most health guidelines also recommend flu shots for people over 65.

Hepatitis B and C Treatments

Both hepatitis B and C are chronic viral diseases that can cause progressive damage to the liver, development of cirrhosis, liver failure, and liver cancer. Both diseases can cause chronic and sometimes profound fatigue in people with mild or no liver damage. In order to eradicate the virus and prevent further damage and regain health, both types require treatment with medication or combinations of medications. Although treatment isn't always successful, when it is, it can stop the progressive damage to the liver and prevent the development of cirrhosis, liver failure, and liver cancer.

Decisions regarding treatment of chronic hepatitis aren't straightforward and can be complex. Each person needs to consider factors together with their medical care provider, such as the potential for disease progression weighed against a prolonged, not always successful, and in some cases (not all) extremely brutal and chemotherapy-like treatment. However, many people who do choose to do treatment and have successful outcomes find that after a period of recovery (which also can be prolonged), they feel much better, their fatigue is gone, and their liver also becomes healthier.

It's a general rule of thumb that 10 percent of people cannot handle the severity of the side effects caused by the treatment and have to discontinue it, 10 percent have little or no side effects, and the remainder of people fall somewhere in between.

Treatment medications for chronic hepatitis C infection are a combination of injectable pegylated *interferon* and oral ribavirin. Treatment medications for chronic hepatitis B infection are a combination of injectable pegylated interferon or interferon-alpha and oral lamivudine, adefovir dipivoxil, entecavir, and telbivudine.

MS Disease-Modifying Medicines

Disease-modifying drugs (DMD) can alter the progression of multiple sclerosis to slow disability by reducing the frequency and severity of relapses. The two types of DMD used in MS are beta *interferon* (has two forms: beta interferon 1a and beta interferon 1b) and glatiramer acetate. They have similar effects but different actions, although they are both based on the idea that MS is an autoimmune disease.

The three types of natural interferon are alpha, beta, and gamma. Alpha interferon is used in cancer and hepatitis treatments but is not thought to be of benefit in treating MS, and gamma interferon has been shown to actually induce MS symptoms. Because

def•i•ni•tion

Interferons are proteins that are produced naturally by the human body and have a vital role in the immune system response to fight off viral infections. Interferon produced by your body is what causes you to feel achy with malaise (sick) during a flulike illness.

beta interferon blocks the action of gamma interferon, it is used to reduce inflammation and the autoimmune reaction that is responsible for the inflammation and destruction of myelin.

Glatiramer acetate mimics the effects of the main proteins in myelin by connecting to cells in the immune system that are thought to switch off inflammation occurring in the central nervous system; this helps the brain and spinal column cells recover.

Experimental Drugs

Ampligen is an antiviral agent that is a synthetic nucleic acid compound (complex compounds found in all living cells and viruses) that works to stimulate the production of interferon in the body. Some believe that using ampligen for CFS may improve cognitive ability and overall physical functioning.

Gamma globulin is an intravenous broad spectrum antibody product derived from pooled human immune globulin that is used to passively immunize people who have been exposed to infectious agents or in people with compromised immune function. Its experimental use in CFS is based on the hypothesis that CFS may be due to an underlying immune disorder.

Growth hormone deficiency in adults has been associated with symptoms seen in CFS and FM such as lack of energy, poor overall health, reduced ability to exercise, muscle weakness, cold intolerance, impaired thinking, unhappiness, sadness and depression, and decreased lean body mass. Fibromyalgia and other chronic disorders such as CFS that are thought to have a blunting of the HPA axis response are also believed by some to possibly have a growth hormone deficiency, and for this reason, CFS doctors like Jacob Teitelbaum prescribe Human Growth Hormone (HGH). Unfortunately, HGH is only FDA approved to promote growth in HGH-deficient children; growth hormone (GH) deficiency syndrome resulting from pituitary disease, surgery, radiation therapy, hypothalamic disease; or injury in adults. It's also expensive and controversial in other uses, such as antiaging or fatigue. It's not likely that your doctor will prescribe HGH unless he is highly specialized in treating CFS and you meet strict criteria.

Over-the-Counter (OTC) Medications

Acetaminophen is used by millions of people to relieve headache pain, joint pain, and muscle pain. Although acetaminophen is thought to be generally safe when taken as recommended, it's important to be aware of all medications you take that contain acetaminophen. Do not take more than four grams or four thousand milligrams in any 24-hour period. Exceeding this maximum dose can lead to liver failure. NSAIDs, including aspirin, ibuprofen, and naprosyn, may be used to relieve pain and fever that is associated with CFS. Follow all manufacturers' instructions and report any adverse effects to your doctor.

OTC antihistamines including diphenhydramine, chlorpheniramine, brompheniramine, clemastine, doxylamine, pseudoephedrine, phenylephrine, oxymetazoline, naphazoline, and pheniramine can be useful in the treatment of allergy symptoms. You can also combine sedating antihistamines such as diphenhydramine with an OTC pain reliever at night to help with insomnia and pain. By using a simple and inexpensive remedy like this, you might avoid the many pitfalls of using prescription sleep and pain medications and still get a good night's sleep.

Body Work

Body work in medicine is a term used to describe therapy or method to improve symptoms typically involving some form of touching, physical work, or manipulation of the body. The following are primary body work methods employed or recommended by medical practitioners:

- **Chiropractic care**—a hands-on, manipulative body work technique used to provide symptom relief in CFS and many other conditions.

- **Osteopathy**—Focuses on the entire musculoskeletal system, not just the spine.

- **Physical therapy**—currently used to treat a wide range of conditions from accidents and injuries to CFS.

- **Rebound exercise**—Done via a physical therapist or at home using a mini-trampoline. It is thought to restore the autonomic nervous system dysfunction in CFS.

- **Hydrotherapy**—Utilizes the significant gradient pressure of water as you float or stand upright in water to the neck.

The premise of chiropractic care is that a lack of vitality and good health are caused by an obstructed flow of nerve impulses from the brain through the spinal nerves to the rest of the body. Misalignments (subluxations) or joint dysfunctions, joint adhesions, and joint fixations interfere with the normal transmission of nerve impulses. Over a period of time, there is pain and impaired function; adjustments done with quick, forceful movements by a chiropractor are thought to change the joint range of movement back to normal so that the flow of normal nerve impulses is restored.

Osteopathy consists of soft tissue stretching, deep tactile pressure, and mobilization or manipulation of joints of the body and cranial work with the bones and membrane attachments in the head. By strengthening the musculoskeletal framework, there are positive effects on your body's nervous, circulatory, and lymphatic systems. Physical therapy is a combination of specific functional training, therapeutic exercise, and the application of heat, cold, ultrasound, and/or electrical stimulation by a trained therapist to relieve symptoms and improve mobility. Because CFS exercise causes you to tire easily, physical therapy can be useful to avoid the ramifications of deconditioning. It can also help with pain, it can decrease range of motion, and help with other issues related to injury and immobility. CFS has been found to have some similarities with the autonomic nervous system problems that were first seen in astronauts. After months in orbit, astronauts lost their autonomic nervous system function that allowed them to stand upright in a gravitational field, so when attempting to exit their capsules, they fainted on standing. This disregulated autonomic condition is similar to that found in CFS. NASA found a way to restore the autonomic nervous system by bouncing the astronauts with a bungee cord type system. This up and down motion is thought to input a wave-like motion into the brain to improve autonomic nervous system tone and function. Rebound exercise can be done via a physical therapist or at home using a minitrampoline.

Energy Bar

Kinetic therapy consists of continuously rotating critically ill patients from side-to-side for purposes of preventing complications such as pneumonia. Using the premises of the bouncing therapy and the idea of kinetics, you can use a rocking chair to simulate the beneficial effects of rebound therapy. This rhythmic motion can help improve autonomic tone in people who are too ill to exercise.

Hydrotherapy utilizes the significant gradient pressure of water as you float or stand upright in water to the neck. This intense water pressure gradient forces tissue lymph into the venous blood system from the thoracic duct, improving symptoms over four to six months of continual therapy. It's thought that the beneficial effects are due to the expanding blood volume and the immune modulating effects of a rapid lymphatic fluid transfusion into your bloodstream with some of it's globulin-like immune effects. Water temperature, time in the water, and frequency of therapy are all factors that might affect the therapeutic response and need to be altered depending on each individual. You can get some of the benefits of hydrotherapy by simply soaking in a warm bath at home.

The Least You Need to Know

◆ Antidepressants can be used to alleviate pain and to improve sleep, energy levels, and cognitive impairment.

◆ A vast array of prescription drugs including benzodiazepines, azapirones, SSRIs, tricyclic antidepressants, MAOIs, risperidone (antipsychotic), beta-blocker drugs, anticonvulsants, narcotic analgesics, muscle relaxants, and tramadol are used for depression, anxiety, extreme pain, Restless Legs Syndrome, and insomnia.

◆ Prescription steroids and OTC anti-inflammatory medications that don't contain cortisone (nonsteroidal anti-inflammatory drugs [NSAIDs]) are used to treat a wide variety of pain.

◆ Successful treatment for hepatitis B and C can decrease the chance for liver cancer and other liver problems.

◆ Disease-modifying drugs (DMD) can alter the progression of multiple sclerosis to slow disability by reducing the frequency and severity of relapses.

◆ Body work includes chiropractic care, osteopathy, physical therapy, rebound exercise, and hydrotherapy.

Chapter 8

Alternative Treatments

In This Chapter

◆ How acupuncture can help

◆ The health benefits of massage

◆ Recommended supplements and herbs

◆ The truth about detoxing

◆ Why, when, and how chelation is useful

Complementary and alternative medicines are products and practices, such as supplements, herbs, acupuncture, and massage, that are not part of standard medical care that you would receive from your doctor.

Traditional Chinese medicine (TCM) is an alternative healing method that looks at ill health in a different way than Western medicine does. Instead of looking at lab tests, Chinese medicine practitioners look at the body and signs and symptoms to determine what is going on within so they can treat the underlying root cause of the illness. Chronic fatigue is seen as a domino in the domino effect, with each problem triggering and compounding others. TCM sees that with prolonged stress on the body, energy flow is disrupted, immune function decreases, the adrenal glands become exhausted, and the central nervous system (CNS) and immune function are disrupted.

This chapter is going to give you an idea of some of the alternative methods you might try for symptom relief. Always discuss any plans you have for using alternative methods first with your doctor as most alternative methods including TCM are not proven by Western medicine as benefiting certain conditions and some may be harmful in some instances.

Acupuncture

Acupuncture is a TCM treatment modality that uses very fine needles inserted into defined acupuncture points or meridians on the body where it's believed that energy freely flows during a healthy state. When this energy is blocked, absent, deficient, excessive, or somehow interrupted, the result is illness or pain. So stimulating the correct point on the meridian releases the energy, called Qi (pronounced *chee*). Using acupuncture along with other TCM treatments such as herbs is ideal to strengthen weakened immune function, nourish blood, increase lymph circulation and natural killer cells, promote the elimination of toxins, and promote deep relaxation.

Acupuncture works on both the central and peripheral nervous systems to release *endorphins*, your body's own pain-control chemicals. It also improves circulation to aid in healing the nervous, endocrine, and immune systems. It is thought to support the adrenal glands which, in turn, helps to relieve adrenal exhaustion and restore energy and balance and regulate other failing body systems.

def•i•ni•tion

Endorphins, your body's natural pain-control chemicals, work to promote relaxation and a sense of well-being, as well as reduce the levels of the stress chemicals cortisol and norepinephrine in your body.

The needles used in acupuncture are very fine and flexible so they do not cause pain. You might feel a slight sensation or sense of electricity at the point of insertion and most likely will find the treatments to be extremely relaxing—you might even fall asleep! By using acupuncture with regular exercise, dietary, and lifestyle changes, many people feel a greater sense of health and well-being within several months.

Massage

Massage is a type of therapy with such great health benefits that hospitals are now using it to aid in healing patients. Massage works directly on the musculoskeletal system to relieve muscle aches and fatigue, and may also work on the nervous system to stimulate the release of endorphins. As a result, your heart rate, respiration, and metabolism slow. Your blood pressure is lowered, which in turn, decreases the harmful effects of stress and relieves pain and muscle tension. Massage is a time-tested form of care used for pain control; the relief of muscle tension, stress, and anxiety; and other profound health benefits. Massage promotes relaxation by easing tense muscles and stiff joints. It improves your sense of health and well-being; and has been shown to help relieve migraine, fibromyalgia, and other pain; it boosts alertness and concentration; increases natural killer cells, which helps your immune function; reduces stress, depression, and anxiety; relieves insomnia; decreases PMS symptoms; and improves the flow of lymph and circulation in the body.

Massage stimulates your blood circulation, improving the oxygen and nutrient supply to your tissues. It also helps to move waste products through the lymphatic system. The following is a review of some types of massage and massage techniques: craniosacral therapy, Swedish massage, lymphatic drainage, deep tissue massage, acupressure, reflexology, and Shiatsu.

Craniosacral massage is a gentle, manual therapy that is thought by some to enhance the body's natural healing processes and is used to treat medical problems associated with pain and dysfunction. This therapy works on the craniosacral system, or the membranes and fluid surrounding and protecting the brain and spinal cord, to improve central nervous system function, remove the negative effects of stress, improve disease resistance, and restore health. Craniosacral massage employs a light touch to the skull to support the natural movement of fluid and to test for restrictions in various parts of the craniosacral system. It's thought that by removing the restriction of fluid, the system can correct itself.

Swedish massage promotes health and well-being by using tapping and shaking motions along with long gliding strokes, kneading, and friction for beneficial effects to nerves, muscles, glands, and circulation.

Lymphatic drainage increases lymphatic circulation to assist in detoxifying and boost energy, improve immune function, relieve stress and depression, and treat injuries. This type of massage is gentle, rhythmic, and deeply relaxing and works to reduce water retention by assisting the movement of lymphatic fluid through the system.

Deep tissue massage reaches the deep portions of muscles and the individual muscle fibers by the use of deep muscle compression and friction. This method is used to release the fibers of the muscles and free toxins and deep-seated tension.

Acupressure is known as acupuncture without needles. Similar to acupuncture, this massage technique uses the meridian points along the energy pathways, but the stimulation is achieved with deep finger pressure instead of needles. The pressure is intended to release energy, reduce stress, and promote harmony and balance to lead to improved health.

Reflexology is an acupressure technique performed at meridian points located on the hands and feet thought to correspond with specific parts of the body. Pressure is applied to tender points believed to correlate with dysfunction to clear out congestion and restore normal functioning.

Shiatsu is the most widely known and used method of acupressure; it uses rhythmic pressure on meridian points with fingers, hands, elbows, knees, and sometimes feet to release and stimulate the flow of energy. This type of therapy can also employ the use of gentle stretching and range-of-motion to treat pain and illness, promote relaxation, and maintain overall health.

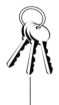

Energy Bar

Defray the cost of regular massages by looking up a local massage therapy school that offers massages from their students at a discount. You also can receive the daily benefit of pain and stress relief by using a portable massage unit. There are many types of units on the market that do all types of massage from acupressure to Shiatsu.

Supplements and Herbs

Supplements are nutrients taken to augment a healthy diet for improvement in illness and disease and for symptom relief. They include vitamins, minerals, herbs, amino acids, enzymes, and other nutrients. If you are taking certain medications such as statins, you need to first consult with your doctor because you may have different recommendations. And always consult with your doctor before taking any supplements, including herbs, because they can interact with your other medications, alter the results of your lab tests, and be toxic in certain doses and combinations. Your doctor may also have more specific recommendations for you based on your personal health history and concerns. And finally remember that supplements never replace a healthy diet—they only help to enhance it!

Vitamins have specific jobs and low levels of a certain vitamin will cause you to have a deficiency disease (for example, an inadequate level of vitamin D leads to a condition known as rickets). It used to be that medics claimed that all supplements did for a person was to cause expensive urine. But today the Standard American Diet (SAD) is typically deficient in the following nutrients: calcium, iron, vitamin A, and vitamin C. Additionally, the recommended daily allowance (RDA) for some nutrients might actually be below what is necessary to offer the best protection to your immune system. For those reasons, more doctors and health-care professionals are now recommending daily vitamin and mineral supplements for optimal health.

Many of the recommended vitamins and minerals can be taken as part of a multivitamin, but some need to be taken separately. Check the label to make sure your supplement provides the recommended daily dose.

Mehmet C. Oz, M.D., cardiac surgeon and coauthor of *YOU On a Diet*, recommends taking the following vitamins and mineral supplements. Note: IU stands for international units, mcg stands for micrograms, and mg stands for milligrams:

- **Vitamin A:** 2,500 IU/day (maximum dose); fat-soluble

- **Pyridoxine (B_6):** 4 mg/day; water-soluble

- **Cobalamin (B_{12}):** 25 mcg/day; water-soluble

- **Vitamin C (ascorbic acid):** 400 mg/day in three divided doses; water-soluble

- **Vitamin D:** 400 IU/day age 59 and under; 600 IU/day age 60 and over; fat-soluble

- **Vitamin E:** 400 to 800 IU/day; fat-soluble

- **Folate (also called folic acid, folate, folicin, or vitamin B_9):** 800 mcg/day; water-soluble

- **Thiamin (B_1):** 25 mg/day; water-soluble

- **Riboflavin (B_2):** 25 mg/day; water-soluble

- **Niacin (B_3):** 30 mg/day; water-soluble

- **Biotin (B_7):** 300 mg/day; water-soluble

- **Pantothenic acid (B_5):** 30 mg/day; water-soluble

- **Calcium:** 1,200 mg/day in two divided doses; because the body uses what it needs and excretes any excess; an essential mineral

- **Magnesium:** 400 mg/day

- **Selenium:** 200 mcg/day

- **Zinc:** 15 mg/day

Jacob Teitelbaum, M.D., is a well-known physician in Annapolis, Maryland, who has studied and written about CFS for decades. According the Dr. Teitelbaum, the "core defect" underlying CFS is a defect in the energy furnaces inside the cell: the mitochondria. The mitochondria produce the energy by way of a chemical called adenosine triphosphate (ATP). When the mitochondria aren't functioning effectively, they don't generate the optimal amount of ATP. Some researchers then aim for supplements that help increase the production of energy in the body as well as those that boost immune function.

If you are suffering from CFS, infections, allergies, and depression, ask your doctor about augmenting your vitamins by adding the following:

- **Malic acid/magnesium hydroxide:** 1,800–6,000 mg in six divided doses; a fruit derived acid that plays an essential role in the production of energy

- **Inositol:** 500 mg/day; also known as vitamin B_8 is a natural sedative thought to regulate the nervous system; water-soluble

- **PABA (para-aminobenzoic acid):** 10 mg/day; a B vitamin important for healthy hair and skin, thought to help prevent damage from pollution and secondhand smoke and reduces inflammation; water-soluble

- **Vitamin C (ascorbic acid):** increase to 2000 mg/day in three divided doses; may increase endurance and immune function; water-soluble

- **Potassium aspartate:** 200 mg/day; may be helpful for fatigue syndromes; is thought to play a role in transporting potassium and magnesium across cell membranes possibly into mitochondria

- **Iron:** 18 mg/day; for iron deficiency anemia only if directed by your doctor

- **Chromium:** 150 mcg/day; a mineral that helps cells break down sugar into energy, thought by some to be deficient in people with CFS

Remember that supplements are not regulated by the FDA and they can't be prescribed to treat any specific medical condition. This means that the claims regarding their health benefits have not been "officially" proven.

Slip-Ups

Don't take your multivitamin capsules all at once. Fat-soluble vitamins need to be taken only once a day because they are stored in the body, whereas water-soluble vitamins need to be taken in divided doses because any excess that isn't immediately needed by the body is excreted in the urine. Buy supplements that direct you to take the capsules two to three times a day. Make sure to take Vitamin B supplements early in the day as they can be stimulating causing insomnia.

Glutathione is a supplement that has been extensively studied but is an unregulated supplement nonetheless. It is a powerful antioxidant that comes in part from the diet but is primarily synthesized in the body and plays a part in nutrient metabolism, DNA and protein synthesis, cell growth, and immune response. Glutathione supplements might not be able to cross the cell membrane and so might not be as effective as eating adequate amounts of fruits and vegetables such as broccoli and brussels sprouts. Spices like cinnamon and cardamom and meats also contain necessary components that are thought to increase glutathione levels.

Stress depletes glutathione as does a chronic toxic load from infections and poisons. Depleted levels can lead to immune dysfunction. Supplementing with other nutrients including alpha lipoic acid, acetylcysteine, methyl donors, and polyphenols such as Pycnogenols help to increase levels of glutathione in the body. Methyl donors include B vitamins, folic acid, TMG, DMG, SAM-e, and DMAE that also help in the production of several brain chemicals to improve mood, energy, well-being, alertness, concentration, and visual clarity.

def•i•ni•tion

Glutathione is an important and powerful antioxidant that works as a free radical scavenger and detoxifier of toxins including heavy metals and pesticides. It also maintains mitochondria (energy-producing cells in the body) and improves immune system function. Glutathione depletion often is associated with CFS.

Methyl donors are substances currently being studied in research regarding cancer and antiaging. They are substances that can transfer a methyl group or a carbon atom attached to three hydrogen atoms to another substance. Yikes! That may be more than you need to know, so suffice it to say that lots of important biochemical processes rely on what is called methylation. Researchers are starting to think that adequate methylation of DNA might stop harmful genes such as cancer genes in their tracks. Antiaging researchers hypothesize that the body's ability to methylate declines with age and contributes to the aging process. In the future we may see more emphasis on methyl donor supplementation based on research.

NAC (N-Acetyl-L-Cysteine) is a precursor to glutathione and thought to improve glutathione stores in your body and to be a powerful immune booster. Recommended doses of NAC typically range from 500–1,200 mg daily.

Alpha lipoic acid is a powerful antioxidant with many uses including protection of the liver; improving diabetic neuropathy, relieving burning mouth syndrome, and other types of nerve pain; and improving glutathione stores. Ask your doctor for advice on dosing as it ranges depending on your problem.

Cod-liver oil is used for treatment of pain as an anti-inflammatory and for treatment of depression and other mood disorders. If you buy capsules, you can freeze them— and when you take the frozen capsules, you aren't as likely to get fish burps later. A typical dose is one half to one tablespoon a day or up to five capsules to supply essential omega-3 fatty acids.

Tyrosine can help relieve depression linked to chronic fatigue. This amino acid is needed by the body to produce the thyroid hormone thyroxine and is made from phenylalanine, another amino acid. Tyrosine typically comes in 750 mg capsules but should be taken in smaller amounts such as 100–200 mg to start as it is overenergizing to some people. Ask your doctor what is best for you.

Phenylalanine is an essential amino acid that must be acquired through diet from fish, poultry, red meat, almonds, lentils, lima beans, chickpeas, and sesame seeds. It can also be taken as a dietary supplement (500–2,000 milligrams per day) and acts as an anti-depressant and pain reliever. Do not take phenylalanine if you are taking monoamine oxidase inhibitor drugs for depression.

Astragalus contains antioxidants and is used to protect and support the immune system, prevent upper respiratory infections and cold, lower blood pressure, treat diabetes, and protect the liver. Astragalus comes in many forms and doses, generally 1–25 mg, depending on whether you are taking dried root, liquid, capsule, etc.

Lavender produces calming, soothing, and sedative effects and is a natural remedy for insomnia, anxiety, depression, and mood disturbances. Used as aromatherapy oil, bath gels, extracts, teas, tincture, and whole dried flowers. Some therapists recommend a drop of the oil on your pillow for a calming effect at night. Other herbs for combating fatigue, stress, and depression and for improving mental and physical capabilities include oat straw, ginger, ginkgo biloba, licorice root, dandelion root, Siberian ginseng, chamomile, hops, catnip, and peppermint teas. Natural anxiety supplements include thiamine (vitamin B₁), 5-HTP, passionflower, valerian, Ashwagandha, trypto-phan, and Skullcap herb. See Appendix C for the link to the University of Maryland's comprehensive website that covers complementary and alternative medicine. It's a thorough source for alternative modalities including information on herbs and supplements.

Siberian ginseng is used to restore vigor, enhance overall health, increase longevity, enhance memory, increase stamina, and stimulate the immune system. It also reduces the frequency, severity, and duration of herpes simplex virus outbreaks.

Ginger and licorice root have been found to boost immunity and strengthen the cardiovascular system. They are powerful antioxidants, improving circulation to the brain, combating fatigue, and boosting adrenal and thyroid gland function. Licorice root should be used only in small amounts because it can lead to potassium loss. Ginger root, ginkgo biloba, licorice root, and dandelion can be taken in a tincture using two droppers-full per day.

Echinacea is a powerful immune stimulant herb that promotes interferon production to help fight infections. It activates natural killer cells (T-lymphocytes) and the cells that kill bacteria (neutrophils). Goldenseal is an immune stimulant that activates the cells that engulf and destroy bacteria, fungi, and viruses (macrophages). Garlic, echinacea, and goldenseal together work well to fend off infections.

Bioflavonoids supplements are very effective in controlling common menopausal symptoms such as hot flashes, anxiety, irritability, and particularly fatigue. Other plant sources of estrogen and progesterone that help alleviate these symptoms include Dong Quai, black cohosh, blue cohosh, unicorn root, false unicorn root, fennel, anise, sarsaparilla, and wild yam root.

Kava kava is useful for alleviating stress, anxiety, depression, and social anxiety. Talk to your doctor if you want to try taking kava because it's not a supplement like vitamin C or B that you take every day. In fact, it is preferable to use kava no more than two times a week because daily use can harm the liver. Kava is, however, recommended by integrative doctors when used as directed. St. John's Wort in low doses works for relieving anxiety within days. GABA is useful for fighting social anxiety and shyness, and SAM-e is used for depression.

The following supplements can be taken to decrease fatigue and improve energy:

◆ **Acetyl-L-Carnitine:** 500 mg. Take it one to two times a day for three months for CFS, FMS, MS, elevated blood triglycerides, and weight loss.

- **Coenzyme Q$_{10}$:** Take 200 mg/day, particularly if you're taking cholesterol-lowering prescriptions. Take it with vitamin E, fatty food, or oil supplements to improve absorption.

- **NADH (Enada):** Take 10 mg sublingual tablets every morning before eating.

- **Panax Ginseng:** Take 100–200 mg twice a day for adrenal fatigue.

- **Ginkgo biloba:** Take 60 mg two to three times a day to help relieve brain fog.

The following supplements have antiviral properties:

- **Monolaurin:** Take 300 mg capsules; nine capsules once a day on an empty stomach for one week, followed by six capsules once a day for three weeks for viral infections.

- **Lysine:** 1,500 mg twice a day to suppress herpes simplex outbreaks.

- **Olive leaf:** Take 1,500 mg three times a day for two weeks for respiratory infections or three times a day for three weeks for chronic viral infections.

Energy Bar

For severe immune dysfunction and fatigue, begin by sipping aloe vera juice and taking peppermint tea, oil in capsules, or tincture. After you gain some strength, begin the other herbs. Oils are prepared entirely with oil, whereas tinctures are prepared using alcohol, which is thought by herbalists to be more easily assimilated by the body.

Natural pain supplements used along with treatments such as massage, acupuncture, stretching, and regular exercise can help alleviate pain while reducing your need for medications that can add to your toxic load and cause additional symptoms related to side effects. Most supplements take time to see the effects, so give them a couple weeks of regular use. The following supplements are useful in pain relief:

- **5-hydroxytryptophan (5-HTP):** Can reduce the number of tender points in people with fibromyalgia, improving symptoms of pain, stiffness, anxiety, fatigue, and sleep.

- **Glucosamine sulfate:** Take 500 mg three times a day for joint health. Glucosamine sulfate actually helps to relieve pain from arthritis. (Recent NIH data shows that it does not repair cartilage, as previously thought. It does, however, relieve pain from arthritis).

- ◆ **Sulfur:** Available in two supplement forms, dimethyl sulfoxide (DMSO) and methylsulfonylmethane (MSM). Both forms are effective treatments for pain. Apply DMSO as a topical analgesic, in a 70 percent DMSO/30 percent water solution. It can take six weeks to take effect but is touted as extremely effective for chronic pain.

- ◆ **MSM (methylsulfonylmethane):** Take 1,000–3,000 mg a day for allergies, wound healing, and arthritis pain. MSM is safe to take even if you are sulfa allergic.

- ◆ **Certo (fruit pectin):** Take one to three tablespoons in eight ounces of grape juice one to two times a day.

- ◆ **Rhus Tox:** Dissolve under the tongue as directed on the bottle and use as needed for muscle pain. Rhus Tox comes in various potencies as tinctures, tablets, and pellets.

- ◆ **Cetyl Myristoleate:** Take three 385-milligram capsules two times a day for 10 days.

- ◆ **Devil's claw:** An herb used for relieving the pain of degenerative joint diseases such as arthritis and low back pain, and as a digestive aid. Your dose is dependant on the form, including capsules, dried tuber or root powder, liquid, tincture, or tea.

- ◆ **Ginger:** Is used fresh or in a powder for body aches, migraines, arthritis pain, and nausea, and to reduce bloating and gas. Your dose is dependant on the form, including fresh or dried root, tablets, capsules, tinctures, and teas.

- ◆ **Dong quai:** An herb that provides relief from menstrual disorders such as cramps, irregular menstrual cycles, infrequent periods, PMS, and menopausal symptoms. Boil the dried herb (raw root) or soak it in wine before consuming. Powdered herb in capsules: 500–600 mg tablets or capsules up to six times daily. Tincture: 40–80 drops three times daily.

- ◆ **Passionflower:** An herb for anxiety and insomnia, it is used to treat pain, insomnia, and nervousness. As a tincture take 10–60 drops, 3 times a day. Infusion (a large amount of herb brewed for a long time) take 2–5 grams of dried herb 3 times a day. As a fluid extract (1:1 in 25 percent alcohol), take 10–30 drops, 3 times a day.

- ◆ **Pau d'arco:** An herb used to treat a wide range of conditions including pain, arthritis, inflammation of the prostate gland (prostatitis), skin lesions, fever, GI upsets, and various cancers. To make tea, use 1 tsp of pau d'arco loose dried bark in 1 cup water, boil for 5–15 minutes. Drink a cup of this 2–8 times a day. Use 20–30 drops of tincture 3 times a day, or take 1,000 mg capsules 3 times a day.

◆ **Peppermint:** An herb taken brewed as tea to soothe anxiety and upset stomachs, or aid in digestion nausea, diarrhea, and flatulence. Peppermint oil also has some antiviral properties. For irritable bowel syndrome, menstrual cramps, or gallstones take 1–2 enteric-coated capsules, 3 times a day, between meals. For itching and skin irritations, apply the active ingredient in peppermint (menthol) in a cream or ointment form not more than 3–4 times per day. For tension headaches, lightly coat the forehead with a tincture of 10 percent peppermint oil to 90 percent ethanol and allow the tincture to evaporate.

◆ **Rosemary:** An herb used to improve memory, relieve muscle pain and spasm, stimulate hair growth, and support the circulatory and nervous systems. Prepare tea by pouring 2 cups boiling water over the 6 grams of herb and steeping for 3–5 minutes. Drink in 3 divided doses over the day. Take as a tincture 2–4 milliliters, 3 times per day. As a wine, add 20 grams of herb to 1 liter of wine and allow to stand for 5 days (shake occasionally). Use the essential oil as purchased in small drops on pillow or in the bath.

◆ **Turmeric:** An anti-inflammatory used to treat digestive disorders and liver problems, and for the treatment of skin diseases and wound healing. Take dried powdered root in capsules of 1,000–3,000 mg per day, as a fluid extract take 30–90 drops a day, or tincture 15–30 drops, 4 times per day.

◆ **Willow bark:** Used for the treatment of pain (particularly lower back pain and osteoarthritis), headache, and inflammatory conditions such as bursitis and tendinitis. The bark of white willow contains salicin, which in the 1800s was used to develop aspirin. For tea, boil 1–2 tsp of dried bark in 8 ounces of water and simmer for 10–15 minutes; let steep for a half hour; drink 3–4 cups per day. Take no more than 60–240 mg of powdered herb per day. Do not use if allergic or sensitive to salicylates (such as aspirin). Take 4–6 milliliters of tincture per day.

◆ **Yarrow:** Used to treat wounds, menstrual ailments, bleeding hemorrhoids, fevers and colds, and stomach and intestinal upset. For tea, pour boiling water over 1–2 teaspoons of dried yarrow, steep for 3–5 minutes. Take 2–4 grams in capsules, 3 times per day; 20–120 drops of extract, 3 times per day; 40–120 drops of tincture, 3 times per day. For a sitz bath, use 3–4 ounces of dried yarrow per 5 gallons of water.

Chelation

Today's world is incredibly toxic. Toxins are in the air we breathe, the water we drink, and the food we consume and are added in tiny FDA-approved amounts to just about every product to improve smell, taste, texture, color, and more. *Chelation* is a medical treatment used for heavy metal poisoning, but you can also detox at home using a systematic approach of good diet and lifestyle measures along with certain supplements.

Small amounts of particular metals such as iron, copper, manganese, and zinc are common in the environment and diet and are essential for good health. However, exposure to large amounts of some metals can cause acute or chronic toxicity. Heavy metal toxicity in the body can happen after long-term and even low-level exposure, most commonly to lead, mercury, arsenic, and cadmium. It's thought that this low-level, long-term exposure to heavy metals might be linked to autoimmune diseases such as CFS, multiple chemical sensitivities (MCS), fibromyalgia, and multiple sclerosis; cardiovascular disease; cognitive difficulties; allergies; and immune system dysfunction.

def•i•ni•tion

Treatment of arsenic, lead, iron, mercury, and aluminum poisoning toxicity includes **chelation** treatment (pronounced key-lay-shun), a process whereby an agent is used to bind and hold molecules of metals or minerals so that they can be removed from the body.

Chronic low-level exposure to toxic heavy metals can come from absorption through the skin; ingestion; or inhalation from sources including aluminum cookware, dental amalgam fillings, tap water, air pollution, cigarette smoke, seafood, pesticides, certain medications, cosmetics, fertilizers, lead paint, and antiperspirants. Levels in the body become toxic when they are not adequately metabolized and they accumulate in the soft tissues.

Symptoms of acute heavy metal toxicity are typically severe, rapid in onset, and strongly associated with the exposure or ingestion. But diagnosing chronic exposure is where it gets tricky because symptoms such as learning difficulties, nervousness, mood swings, insomnia, nausea, fatigue, and not feeling well develop over time and are very similar to symptoms of other health conditions. The symptoms can also come and go, so the causal link is often undefined and an ill person might put off seeking treatment.

If you suspect that you have heavy metal toxicity, partner with your physician in initiating an appropriate workup. The diagnosis of heavy metal toxicity requires a thorough history of any potential exposure, including occupation, hobbies, recreational activities, environment, correlating symptoms, and laboratory tests (including blood tests, urinalysis, fecal tests, x-rays, and hair and fingernail analysis). Most professionals administer chelation therapy in consultation with a poison control center or a medical toxicologist and along with other supportive measures depending on the severity of the poisoning.

Chelation therapy can include a programmed series of intravenous infusions, intra-muscular injections, or oral administration of a chelating agent. A combination of the three over a few hours to several days of inpatient treatment also can be administered. Some people require repeated courses, and follow-up testing is necessary to check the amount of the metal being removed.

Ethylene diamine tetraacetic acid (EDTA) has been approved by the FDA as a chelat-ing agent for lead, mercury, or arsenic poisoning. It is delivered through an intravenous injection typically with vitamins and minerals (such as vitamin C and magnesium) because, along with pulling out heavy metals, the chelating agent also pulls out nutri-ents from the bloodstream.

Detoxing

Common signs and symptoms of environmental toxicity include memory loss, acne, rashes, headaches, aches and pains, fertility problems, fatigue, muscle weakness, tinni-tus, and immune system dysfunction. Detoxing is a systematic approach that includes raising your awareness of possible toxins; avoiding toxins including caffeine, MSG, sugar, aspartame, Splenda, smoking, and drugs; and removing toxins from your diet and environment.

Aluminum is not a heavy metal, but it's the third most abundant element on earth and commonly found in food additives, antacids, buffered aspirin, astringents, nasal sprays, antiperspirants, and drinking water; it is used to make foil, cookware, cans, ceramics, and fireworks. Aluminum has been studied and causally linked to Alzheimer's dis-ease. Although it might not be a primary cause, a majority of researchers agree it's an important factor in Alzheimer's. Aluminum can affect the central nervous system, kid-neys, and digestive system, but there are no recommendations from the FDA against using aluminum-containing products, so limiting your exposure is a personal decision.

In the case of any suspected mercury toxicity, the first and most important step is to remove the source of mercury by having dental amalgams removed and avoiding eat-ing contaminated fish. Find a dentist who is properly trained to remove your amal-gams because improper removal is thought by some to result in additional exposure to mercury.

Detox diets and protocols have seen a recent popularity, but the truth is that toxins—including heavy metals—are stored in fat and the process of detoxing takes place over time, not just a week or a month like some detox protocols claim. Also, detoxification needs a lot of supplied energy to reduce the metabolic burden on the body, so protocols that consist largely of water or juice fasts do not supply the necessary essential nutrients required for healthy detoxification. Water, juice, or fast-type detox protocols cause you to break down your lean tissue instead of fat for energy and only increase harmful free radicals in your body.

In The Know

"I think that physicians are generally uneducated in the whole realm of lifestyle medicine—that is, how diet, exercise, mental states, and habits all affect health. I think they're very uneducated in mind-body interactions and the spiritual dimension of human health. I think there's almost a complete omission of education about nutrition, about use of dietary supplements, about use of botanicals, about many of these other systems of medicine, like Ayurvedic and Chinese medicine, which are thousands of years old and very effective in many areas. So there are large areas, I think, of omission in conventional medical education.

—*Andrew Weil, M.D., internationally recognized expert on integrative medicine*

Diets rich in or supplemented with vitamins, minerals, amino acids, and herbs that are beneficial, protective, and supportive of good health will give you ongoing detoxification using your body's own inherent chelation mechanisms. Detoxing is a continual, unending process taking place within the liver, kidneys, intestines, lymph, blood, and every cell in the body.

A detox diet supplemented with foods that are known to help mobilize and excrete toxins is a good way to kick off your lifetime of good eating habits. This sort of detox diet launching pad should include high-energy macronutrients (protein, fat, and carbs) with "low-allergy-potential." Include high-quality protein to help eliminate toxic metal, olive oil to protect against chemically induced liver damage, and fiber to support fecal excretion of toxins and intestinal health (thereby decreasing your toxic burden). Rice bran from eating brown rice actually binds some toxins so that they are not absorbed but are excreted before they can enter the body. This is another illustration of why a varied, well-balanced daily diet of real whole food is important for optimal health.

The following nutrients and phytonutrients in the diet are thought to be helpful for detoxification of toxins and heavy metals by some practitioners in the wellness/ integrative medicine community (although many dietary and nutritional claims may not be backed up by what is known as hard science):

◆ Alfalfa is an exceptional source of protein and high in vitamins A, D, E, B_6, and K; calcium; magnesium; chlorophyll; phosphorus; iron; potassium; trace minerals; and several digestive enzymes. Alfalfa is also a high-fiber substance with properties that bind and remove toxins from the colon. Don't take alfalfa if you have iron overload.

◆ Alpha lipoic acid is a potent antioxidant that increases production of glutathione in the body helping to dissolve toxins in the liver. Alpha lipoic acid has been used in the treatment of liver and heart disease, diabetes, and other inflammatory diseases.

◆ Artichoke is a liver protectant and antioxidant that can decrease the loss of *glutathione* after toxic exposure.

◆ Bioflavonoids are antioxidants that naturally bond with and remove metals from the body.

◆ Catechins from green tea are strong antioxidants that inhibit the growth of cancer cells, improve the ratio of good (HDL) cholesterol to bad (LDL) cholesterol, are associated with lower incidence of Parkinson's disease, enhance immune function, and promote healthy gastrointestinal function.

◆ Chlorella is a green algae super food that enhances the immune system. It appears to bind to heavy metals as well as other toxic substances such as dioxin and polychlorinated biphenyls (PCBs—chemical compounds found in plastics, insulation, and flame-retardants that may have links to cancer and liver damage) in the bowel and helps with the detoxification process. Some dentists recommend chlorella when patients are having mercury amalgams removed.

◆ Cilantro works as a chelator to move mercury, aluminum, and lead out of the central nervous system so that it can be more easily removed. Taking cilantro four times a day for two to three weeks will help to remove any mercury deposits in your body after you have dental amalgams removed.

◆ Ellagic acid (from pomegranate) can protect against cancers, protects from toxin liver damage, enhances glutathione production, and binds some metals promoting their excretion.

◆ Garlic protects you from various pollutants and heavy metals and prevents certain kinds of cancer.

◆ N-acetylcysteine increases serum sulfate levels to support glutathione production for balanced, complete detoxification. Take 200–500 mg per day.

◆ Rutin is a plant extract found in buckwheat, black tea, and apple peel. It has antioxidant, anti-inflammatory, and anticarcinogenic properties and helps to chelate iron.

◆ Selenium and zinc are antioxidants that enhance immune system function and protect the body against the effects of stress, including chemotherapy.

◆ Silymarin from milk thistle increases synthesis of glutathione, is a strong antioxidant, and can improve liver function in patients with liver disease and toxicity. Milk thistle's role in heavy metal detoxification is its ability to aid liver function and regeneration.

◆ Vitamin B_1 (thiamin), vitamin B_2 (riboflavin), vitamin B_3 (niacin), vitamin B_5 (pantothenic acid), and magnesium are necessary to support energy production.

◆ Vitamin B_{12} (cobalamin), folate, methionine, and choline promote balanced detoxification.

◆ Vitamin C (ascorbic acid) helps to mobilize and detoxify lead, mercury, and chemical poisons.

◆ Watercress has components that can inhibit the growth of cancer cells and promote the excretion of carcinogens.

The Least You Need to Know

◆ Acupuncture, along with an exercise program and dietary and lifestyle changes, is a useful treatment for fatigue and restoring health and balance.

◆ There are many different massage techniques, all with varied health benefits including home units that will give you daily pain and stress relief.

◆ Supplements and herbs augment a healthy diet and are used to improve health, treat illness, and alleviate symptoms of illness and fatigue.

◆ Chelation is a process used to pull toxic heavy metals that are associated with many health conditions out of that body.

◆ Detoxing is an ongoing process that takes place in your body. You become aware of sources of toxins, avoid and limit your exposure to toxins, and remove toxins from your diet and environment. A detox diet augmented with certain foods and supplements can help you to launch a lifetime of good eating habits.

Psychological Healing

In This Chapter

- ◆ Another way to measure fatigue impact
- ◆ Professionals you can lean on
- ◆ Measures to try at home
- ◆ Are medications causing your fatigue?

You might be dealing with psychological stressors, like anxiety and depression, which are causing or worsening your fatigue. If you have significant depression or anxiety it's imperative you see a doctor right away and follow their recommended treatment plan that may include both medications and counseling.

As you continue to read, you will see that there is not just one magic bullet remedy for fatigue. Instead, it's a combination of addressing each fatigue stressor in your life and changing unhealthy behaviors. That said, it follows that researchers have found that it isn't just therapy that improves fatigue in patients with cancer, for example—it's therapy combined with exercise! It makes sense that you get the best results when you have a diverse game plan.

Your psychological healing can come from a variety of sources, including counseling; educating yourself (information is power); psychotherapy; medications; self-help groups and support groups; group psychotherapy; anxiety management; behavior therapy; hypnosis; and the many self-help, mind-body, stress, and relaxation techniques outlined in this book.

How Bad Is It?

Even though fatigue might have taken a huge toll, it might not be easy for you to quantify its effects on your life to others or even yourself. Because fatigue has such a huge impact on your quality of life, many researchers have studied how to measure the subjective experience of fatigue to better understand your level of impairment. The Fatigue Severity Scale (FSS) is a widely used method developed by Lauren Krupp, M.D., professor of neurology and psychology at the State University of New York at Stony Brook and Medical Center, whose specialty is multiple sclerosis (MS). The FSS is a short questionnaire with which you can rate your level of fatigue.

Take the following test and give each statement a number on a scale from one (indicating your strong disagreement) to seven (indicating your strong agreement).

During the past week, I have found that:

◆ My motivation is lower when I am fatigued.

◆ Exercise brings on my fatigue.

◆ I am easily fatigued.

◆ Fatigue interferes with my physical functioning.

◆ Fatigue causes frequent problems for me.

◆ My fatigue prevents sustained physical functioning.

◆ Fatigue interferes with carrying out certain duties and responsibilities.

◆ Fatigue is among my three most disabling symptoms.

◆ Fatigue interferes with my work, family, or social life.

Add up your score for all the statements. A score of 36 or less suggests that you might not be suffering from fatigue, whereas a score higher than 36 indicates that fatigue has a significant impact on your life. You can share this information with a therapist, counselor, or anyone else, for that matter, who you would like to have better understand what you are going through.

Therapy and Counseling

Undergoing psychotherapy can help to improve your fatigue because your therapist will have a bird's-eye view of what might be behind some of your behaviors and destructive ways of thinking. And if you have a very severe fatigue state like Chronic Fatigue Syndrome (CFS), you might need someone to help you cope with your new limitations and the fears that a chronic condition can bring.

You can find the help you need from a variety of sources. A licensed clinical psychologist, clinical social worker, marriage and family therapist, or psychiatrist can conduct the necessary therapy. Unlicensed counselors also might be a good source of therapy, as would a pastor at your church. In therapy, you can look into your feelings about your situation, recognize problems in relating within your family, and learn how to manage your symptoms and the challenges you might have coping with how the stressors might have caused or worsened your fatigue. It has been well proven that therapy can be as effective as antidepressant medication and that therapy used in conjunction with medication is usually more effective and long-lasting for the treatment of depression.

Slip-Ups

Don't continue to eat food made with enriched white flour, sugar, refined cereals, and other junk and processed foods, or drink an excess of tea, coffee, and sodas (diet and otherwise) and expect counseling to do it all. Chances are, if you begin to adequately feed your brain and body while you are working on your issues, you're going to see dramatic improvements in all areas of your life.

If you are having difficulty coping and find that your life is even more stressful, therapy can help you to readjust your life and understand that this time is transitory while giving you the support to accept some of the changes. It's not uncommon when you have a symptom like fatigue to become very down on yourself and internalize feelings such as "being a loser" because you can't do the things you used to do, even if those things were unhealthy behaviors that caused you to get this way in the first place.

If you have severe fatigue such as CFS, you have even more internal challenges because of the high degree of your disability, but the world in general doesn't usually see it or understand it. The more severe your fatigue, the greater the difficulty to cope, accept, adjust, and learn to be patient. Psychotherapy and counseling can improve the quality of your life and give you someone to help you be accountable to in carrying out your self-help work outlined in this book. An objective person also will assist you in seeing your circumstances in the right perspective and keep you from being mired in a state of constant despair or fear.

Cognitive-Behavioral Therapy

Cognitive-Behavioral Therapy (CBT) is a widely accepted, studied, and proven treatment that focuses on changing patterns of faulty thinking and the beliefs that support this unhealthy and distorted thinking. For example, you might be thinking "I'm a loser," and while you might have strong convictions and reasons to support that thinking, a therapist can help you to see how this thought is simply an assumption rather than a fact.

CBT uses methods to help you monitor thoughts that pop into your head, called "automatic thoughts," so you can see the patterns of distorted thinking you have and begin to acquire more healthy alternatives to your thoughts. In CBT your therapist will generally be problem-focused, active, and goal-directed.

This type of therapy is based on the premise that it's your thoughts that actually cause your feelings and behaviors rather than external events and people. And so by changing the way you think, you can feel and behave better even if your situation doesn't change. CBT is thought to have relatively quick results in relation to other sorts of therapy such as psychoanalysis, typically averaging 16 sessions to achieve success in learning and adopting the various problem-solving approaches involved. And unlike psychotherapy, CBT is not open-ended. Rather, you and the therapist understand that it has a specific time frame where you will together decide when you've reached your goal or goals and the therapy will end.

In The Know

"While the results (of CBT trials) support the role of beliefs in maintaining illness in CFS, this does not mean that CFS is necessarily psychological in origin. For instance, CBT can improve the symptoms of patients with other chronic diseases such as rheumatoid arthritis."

—Dr. Benjamin H. Natelson, Department of Neurosciences, New Jersey Medical School

---

Remember that CBT is not psychoanalysis and you don't have to go through delving into your dreams, childhood, or subconscious. Instead, your therapist will help you formulate goals and coach you on how to reach them. It's not about just thinking positively either; it's about reprogramming your mind to think accurately.

Although you might feel that you've lost control over your life, CBT can assist you in recognizing the ways in which you really are in control. And you can begin to use that strength to refocus your passions into healthy behaviors instead of continually convincing yourself that the worst-case scenarios are true. Some people have known for centuries the power that thinking has on our lives. Marcus Aurelius Antoninus (121–180 C.E.), Roman emperor and philosopher, said, "The universe is change; our life is what our thoughts make it."

CBT has been proven to be as useful as antidepressant medication for depression and also better at preventing relapses. It's used as a treatment for anxiety disorders, obsessions, compulsions, and phobias including social phobia. And because the focus of CBT is on thoughts and beliefs, this therapy is applicable and useful for a wide array of issues. If you think this therapy would help you, be sure to ask your therapist what CBT training he has had or contact a Center for Cognitive Therapy and request a referral.

Self-Help and Support Groups

Self-help and support groups are great ways to improve your self-esteem and adopt healthier lifestyle habits. Some groups are led by licensed professional therapists and are generally organized around teaching specific skills, depending on the nature of the group. If you are attending a chronic fatigue or chronic illness group, you might learn skills that include meditation and relaxation, visualization, pain control, stress reduction, and other coping techniques. Support groups also give you the benefit of a "we are in this together" mentality and an avenue to pay it forward by helping others with the benefit of your expertise or such things as offering insights you've had along the way.

def•i•ni•tion

Self-help groups are voluntary meetings for people to share about a common problem or condition. Members have the opportunity to offer ideas and support on issues such as how to cope, heal, improve the quality of their lives, and move forward. Self-help groups are typically free of charge, open to new members, and have ongoing meetings at specific times on certain days of the week.

Group therapy can help you deal with the stress of how your life has been affected and avoid becoming isolated. You can receive validation of your feelings from others who are going through the same thing you are and help you to recognize such things as your limitations and how to effectively deal with them. Often, someone who has walked a mile in your shoes can be much more helpful to you than a professional who you might feel doesn't really understand where you are coming from.

There are some things to watch for and to be aware of in self-help support groups. Don't fall prey to a group that is only supporting being a victim and not supporting behaviors that will move you and the rest of the group forward. Even though you are all there for each other, be aware of groups in which one or more members feel they need to continually slog through how much they are suffering.

It's okay to agree that you are all going through difficult times, but it's not okay for members to belabor every ailment they have or to talk at length about futile subjects. In other words, you don't want to be part of a group that is wearing their predicament as a badge of honor or that gives you the feeling that you have to succumb to defeat. Rather, identify and change the group's dynamics or move on to a healthier group. The ideal group is one that discusses healing methods and how these methods are working for them. An unhealthy group is one that talks about how bad things are for them where people sit around exchanging their horror stories and doom and gloom.

You don't have to go to a professional group to get the benefits of group therapy, though. Rather, you can attend informal groups that are often advertised in newspapers, online, or at your church. If you can't find a group you feel meets your needs, start a group in your own home. The benefit of having your own group is that you can structure it for your own personal needs and attract others who have the same desires, and even values. Possible groups might be recovering addicts, health-oriented groups, runners, vegetarians, or religious or church groups centered on overcoming certain issues.

Guided Imagery/Visualization

Some therapists might help you use the technique of *visualization* or *guided imagery* to help you imagine, think, or visualize how you want your condition to improve over time. You can try this technique by yourself at home!

Imagery involves visualizing your immune system as healthy and balanced, working to fend off viruses and other invaders, an efficient healing force to overcome any condition. Visualization is a process in which you can experience relief of pain; speed the healing process; and help your body to overcome depression, allergies, and many other conditions.

def•i•ni•tion

Visualization or **guided imagery** is an alternative medicine technique where you use your imagination to visualize improved health by "attacking" a disease or health problem in your mind. By using certain meditation-like steps, you use positive thinking to believe you effect healing and disease outcome. This technique is now utilized as "complimentary medicine" in some medical facilities, including oncology centers.

It's thought that any message we send through the conduits that connect mind and body somehow influence what goes on at the cellular level, so the body ultimately responds to our orders. Many experts in using this technique feel that those who are sick might be inadvertently instructing their bodies to stay that way. The following outlines the basic steps in visualization:

1. Determine what you want to work on or your intention (healing your body, a problem such as anxiety). Your intention should be clear, specific, achievable, and you should feel, trust, and know it is being accomplished. What you believe is what your body will do.

2. Find a quiet place to relax lying down or sitting in a comfortable chair.

3. Loosen clothing and get comfortable. Uncross your arms and legs. Center yourself by focusing on breathing.

4. Banish any intruding thoughts by thinking or speaking of your intended area of healing.

5. Close your eyes and envision yourself in the place you want to be in the area of healing. (Imagine being in a very beautiful place happy and healthy.) Visualize yourself as healthy and whole, watching as your body heals you. (Watch the cells in your body and immune system fight off invaders, see your pain flying away.)

6. Feel the sensation of healing. Trust and believe that healing is taking place.

You can pick up visualization books or tapes to help you learn and practice and you can make a tape of yourself to help guide you through each session.

Some studies have illustrated how people can suppress their inflammatory reactions and white cell response to disease-producing organisms or can alternatively allow the inflammatory reaction to respond to normally boost immune function.

It's thought that by imagining a healthy immune system, brain, and adrenal function, for example, people can influence their health and improve immunity by exerting their inner control. In studies of the blood of people who are practicing imagery, this actually has been illustrated by improvements in immune functions such as increases in natural killer cell activity.

Art therapy is another way to use imagery in healing. Art therapists are skilled professionals who help you unleash your internal imagery on paper, canvas, sculpture, or other art media. You can use the power of imagery on your own by drawing. Drawings can help you to first reveal your inner attitudes and beliefs about your circumstances so you understand more clearly your internal struggle. You might, at first, draw yourself tied up or in prison. You can then start making drawings that depict freedom and strengths, like drawing yourself with wings and flying.

Imagery and visualization will help you to believe that you can recover and feel well. And believing is absolutely essential to heal, particularly if you have severe fatigue like CFS. If you never see yourself well, chances are you might just succumb to defeat and not put the effort you need to in order to do the healing work.

To start your visualization program, begin by using some relaxation techniques and deep breathing. As you become relaxed, begin to focus your attention on your internal imagery. For example, if you are experiencing a lot of nausea or GI distress, you might picture your stomach looking like a piece of bloody chuck steak. You can then change that image to something healing, like cool water running over smooth rocks.

Then see yourself as completely healed and engaged in something you love to do, such as hiking in a beautiful meadow. Imagine the internal high you experience with those sorts of activities.

It doesn't matter what you choose to imagine as the healing force inside your body. You can have little soldiers or daggers running through your bloodstream to eradicate invaders, but the outcome in your visualization needs to be focused on a healed you. Incorporate a healthy-looking you that is in better physical shape with better habits and behaviors.

Try to practice imagery three times a day for a few minutes a day. The end point of your visualization always needs to be the best-case scenario of the healthy recovered person you intend to be after you have implemented all the healing behaviors and techniques and you are overflowing with health.

Neurotherapy

Neurotherapy, also called electroencephalograph (EEG) biofeedback and neurofeedback, is a painless and noninvasive treatment approach that allows you to learn about your abnormal brain wave activity to change it. This form of treatment has been shown to improve symptoms of depression, memory and concentration problems, sleep disturbances, cognitive deficits, chronic pain including headaches that are typical of CFS and FM, and many more conditions not listed here.

To undergo neurotherapy, you are connected to EEG equipment with sensors placed on your scalp and ears. You then observe your brain wave activity on a computer monitor as a neurotherapy practitioner helps you learn to change your brain wave activity while you play a computerized video game using your own brain waves. Some of the games are similar to *Pac-Man*, where you move a figure by producing specific brain wave patterns. When you produce the correct brain wave activity, you are able to see it because you move the figure through the maze correctly. In this way, you learn to change abnormal brain wave activity.

Your brain generates four types of brain waves, typically in a mixture of frequencies during a given time with a dominant frequency that varies depending on your state of consciousness. Beta waves are the fastest waves followed by alpha, theta, and delta in that order. Your normal waking state consists principally of beta waves in your brain. When you close your eyes and begin to relax, your brain produces alpha waves followed by a brief period of theta, and then delta when you are asleep. There are many reasons you might have faulty brain waves, including injuries that can cause your brain to produce too much theta or delta waves during times at which you are supposed to be awake and alert.

In The Know

"A neurofeedback protocol in which CFS subjects are trained to increase alpha frequency and power with eyes closed, and reduce the amount of lower frequency EEG activity might prove to be successful in reducing at least some of the symptomology associated with this disorder."

—"EEG Patterns and Chronic Fatigue Syndrome," by Katherine M. Billiot, M.A., Thomas H. Budzynski, Ph.D., and Frank Andrasik, Ph.D.

With neurotherapy, you can learn to change your abnormal brain waves so you can get the restorative sleep that you need and experience enormous improvements in your overall health. In other words, this EEG training can reboot your brain so your brain's regulation of its activity will be restored to more normal ranges.

Some reported side effects of neurotherapy treatments are headaches, anxiety, frustration, fatigue, dizziness, and tingling sensations, but they are usually transient if they do happen at all. The treatment itself is tiring because it's a lot of work, but the benefits outweigh the short-term fatigue the treatment can cause.

To begin, you need to go through an evaluation process that involves a quantitative EEG (qEEG), also called brain mapping, done by a Biofeedback Certification Institute of America (BCIA) certified EEG professional. If you have CFS, you then can evaluate the effectiveness of neurotherapy by trying a sequence of 10 short, generally half-hour sessions that are conducted at least three times a week. By that time, if you don't see a change in your sleep patterns or a reduction in fatigue and pain, you might not be experiencing symptoms caused by abnormal brain waves. If you do see a difference, you can continue on with the treatment. Normally, brain wave training consists of one to three training sessions per week for a total of forty or more sessions over a period of several months.

When you are looking for a neurotherapist, chose a professional who is certified in the use of EEG biofeedback, a licensed health-care practitioner who also does neurotherapy, or someone who is certified and licensed.

You can find a qualified practitioner and get answers by contacting The Biofeedback Certification Institute of America by e-mail at bcia@resourcenter.com.

Online Forums

Internet forums are a twenty-first-century phenomenon. They started around 1996 and are changing the way people relate, communicate, learn, and grow. They are simply groups for having discussions and posting information relevant to the group's purpose using a web application or software. Internet forums are known as message boards, web forums, electronic discussion boards and groups, and forums. Within the forum, you will find topics and subtopics where discussions are taking place. Participants can write comments, ask questions, or offer support to others taking part in the thread (one post after another).

When you frequent an online community, you meet new friends from all around the world and develop a sense of virtual community with the regular users. A huge number of forums exist for an endless number of topics.

The benefits of joining forums are infinite, including friendship and support; you also have the benefit of being able to connect with others at any hour and without having to get dressed and drive someplace. Credible forums do not tout any sort of cures or give medical information even though their purpose may be a support group for a medical condition. If you notice someone "playing doctor," giving medical advice, either bring it up to the group or move on. Do not take any advice from the Internet in regard to medical treatment including recommendations for supplements, herbs, or any other remedy without talking to your doctor.

Are Medications Causing Your Fatigue?

Lots of different prescription and nonprescription medicines have the potential to cause generalized weakness and fatigue that will vary from person to person. Some of these medications include the following:

- Antianxiety medications or tranquilizers
- Antihistamines
- High blood pressure medicines
- Diuretics
- Pain medicine, muscle relaxants
- Steroids
- Tricyclic antidepressants
- Statins
- Birth control pills

Talk to your doctor if you think a prescription or nonprescription medicine may be causing your fatigue or problems such as weakness. You might not realize that OTC medications including pain relievers, cough and cold medicines, antihistamines and allergy medicines, sleeping pills, and motion sickness pills have been inadvertently robbing you of energy. Or you may have been prescribed tranquilizers, antidepressants, muscle relaxants, sedatives, birth control, and blood pressure medication at some point and you feel you don't need them. (You've lost weight; you don't feel depressed; your pain has resolved.) That's when it's time to talk to your doctor about your game plan for reducing, tapering, or just stopping a medication.

Medication, even those that may cause fatigue, are at times necessary. But often, a different medication exists you and your doctor may try that won't cause you to feel fatigued.

In some cases you may find yourself having a problem with certain medications, which include tolerance, dependence, or even addiction. If you think that you don't need a medication anymore but you find yourself worried about stopping it, that's when it's time to have a heart-to-heart talk with your doctor. Talking about your concerns will do a lot to alleviate any emotional distress you may have. Talk to your doctor about how to discontinue your problem medication in a safe and intelligent way. Chances are he or she will be happy to work with you if the condition that you originally took the medication for is resolved.

That said, you shouldn't ever be forced to discontinue a medication against your will that you were encouraged to take. The process for discontinuing a medication will differ for each individual and for each medication. Some doctors are better versed than others in tapering schedules of medications such as antianxiety drugs and antidepressants. If you uncomfortable with the schedule for tapering your doctor has outlined for you, then find a doctor you can work with. Most people who want to come off can come off such medications as antidepressants and benzodiazepines successfully without adverse symptoms and distress.

In The Know

"One of the most difficult aspects of tapering antidepressants is how widely patients vary in their susceptibility to withdrawal reactions. While one patient might be able to taper off an antidepressant in two months, the next patient might need to take eight months to taper off the same dose of the same antidepressant."

—Joseph Glenmullen, M.D., clinical instructor of psychiatry, Harvard Medical School

---

Having adequate psychological support from your spouse, partner, family, friends, an understanding doctor, psychologist, counselor, or other therapist is going to help you succeed. Someone to help you with and to enforce relaxation techniques and deep breathing, or to work with you using alternative techniques such as aromatherapy, acupuncture, or yoga, will also be beneficial as you go along.

If you need to, get help from psychotherapy, and time your taper during a time of low stress. Be sure to exercise regularly, eat a whole food and balanced diet, check that your hormones are balanced and are being treated for imbalances like hypothyroid, take any necessary supplements, and have a strong support system.

The Least You Need to Know

◆ The Fatigue Severity Scale is a widely used method using a short questionnaire on which you can rate your level of fatigue.

◆ Therapy can be conducted by a licensed clinical psychologist, clinical social worker, marriage and family therapist, or psychiatrist.

◆ Cognitive-Behavioral Therapy is a proven treatment that focuses on changing the patterns of faulty thinking and the beliefs that support this unhealthy and distorted thinking.

◆ Self-help and support groups, and Internet forums are a great way to improve your self-esteem, get validation and support, and adopt healthier lifestyle habits.

◆ You can use imagery or visualization to imagine a healthy immune system, brain, and adrenal function to influence your health and improve immunity by exerting your inner control.

◆ Neurotherapy is a painless and noninvasive treatment approach that allows you to learn about your abnormal brain wave activity to change it and improve symptoms of depression, memory and concentration problems, sleep disturbances, cognitive deficits, chronic pain, and many more conditions.

Part 3

Taking Care of Yourself

You can't just pull out one weed to have a weed-free garden; you need to get them all. That same principle applies to overcoming fatigue. No one is exempt from the laws of physiology—everyone needs nutrients, rest, exercise, and fun—and to cultivate health you need to pull out those toxic ways and sow healthy seeds of behavior and lifestyle habits.

In this part, you'll learn the basics of nutrition; the importance of rest, relaxation, and fun; what self-care is; the importance of staying positive; and ways to feel "up" even when you're feeling bad. You'll learn how to refocus your energy so you can not only say good-bye to fatigue, but also reboot into a better, healthier, more productive life.

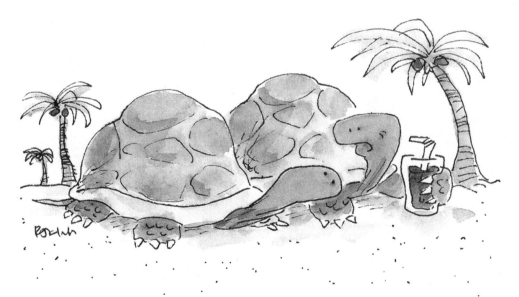

"This smoothie every morning has really given me a lot of pep."

Chapter 10

Let Food Be Your Medicine

In This Chapter

- ◆ Why you need to eat real food to heal
- ◆ The role of nutrients in health and immune function
- ◆ Keeping your blood sugar steady
- ◆ When to eat
- ◆ Pointers for eating well

Nearly 2,500 years ago Hippocrates understood how diet related to healing when he said, "Food should be our medicine and our medicine should be our food" and "Leave your drugs in the chemist's pot if you can heal the patient with food." But we are just beginning to understand and accept that there is a strong relationship between nutrition and immune function.

With the continual bombardment from the media, magazines, and health and diet books galore on food, it's hard to decipher the hype from reality about one of the most basic things we do: eating! This chapter is going to give you a basic rundown on food and nutrition and why it's important to eat right to live; grow; stay healthy and feel well; get energy we need; defend; heal; and recover from stressors such as pressures of life, injuries, and common illnesses.

What Is Real Food?

You probably are wondering what makes real food different from any other food. Food is food, right? Wrong.

Real food can be identified as something that was growing and alive at one time, it spoils, it usually requires some sort of preparation, it has flavor specific to its species, and it has varied colors and textures specific to its type.

A diet of real whole food consists of meals and snacks that are prepared using produce, dairy, meat, fish, nuts, whole grains, oils, legumes, and seeds. A wide variety of real whole food in the proper ratio of fat, protein, and carbohydrates provides the body with the beneficial vitamins, minerals, and nutrients it needs to stay healthy.

Processed foods, on the other hand, might or might not have been alive at one point, it usually doesn't spoil, it is often already prepared, it just has to be taken out of its wrapper to be consumed, and the flavor usually is created in the lab. Also, processed, junk, and convenience foods have a strong link to obesity and degenerative diseases.

You might not realize that eating processed food and drinking soda—even diet soda—can trigger hunger because the sugar and some of the chemicals used in these products actually work on the brain to make you crave more. Many processed foods also don't give your body that signal of satiety. Whole real food, on the other hand, contains the kind of fats, protein, and carbohydrates that your body recognizes to make you feel full and satisfied.

Why Proper Nutrition Is Essential

You see the terms everywhere, on cereal boxes, bread bags, and orange juice containers: "contains vitamins and minerals." But what are they, and what do they have to do with proper nutrition and fighting fatigue?

Getting the proper vitamins and minerals, also known as *nutrients*, gives your body a critical edge in fighting fatigue, illness, and disease. Your body has an inherent ability to heal thanks to these important components of healing.

On the other hand, nutritional deficiencies in the diet can weaken the immune system leading to fatigue or a lack of well-being, mental health issues, decreased resistance to disease and infection, and a slower recovery from all stressors including injury and surgery.

Our bodies need this edge because there are attackers all around. Free radicals are toxic by-products our bodies make continually during metabolic processes regardless of what kind of food a person eats. They come from processed foods and cooking oils that are manufactured with heat because both heat and light damages the delicate oils. That's why experts recommend using oils that don't require heat to process such as coconut, walnut, and olive oil. They also are by-products of cigarette smoke, pollution, sunlight exposure, and other environmental toxins.

Free radicals damage DNA; suppress the immune system; accelerate aging; and have strong links to diseases such as cancer, heart disease, and diseases of the central nervous system, kidney, gastrointestinal, and skin.

> **In The Know**
>
> "We are entering a new era in preventive medicine, which focuses on diet as a means to health."
>
> —Mark Lucock Ph.D., British Medical Journal

Antioxidants, on the other hand, are vitamins and minerals in food that work to remove harmful oxidants or free radicals from the body. Research tells us that diets high in antioxidants help protect against disease, but you can't prevent disease simply by taking supplements. You need to eat a diet of a variety of real whole foods with all their synergist components; supplements only augment a good diet, they don't replace it.

Ideally, your meals and snacks need a ratio of about 40 percent carbohydrates, 30 percent protein, and 30 percent fat. By eating this balance, you are getting the right amounts of *macronutrients* and *micronutrients* necessary for metabolic processes every time you eat.

def•i•ni•tion

Vitamins, minerals, and phytonutrients are known as **micronutrients** because they are needed in relatively small amounts in comparison to the **macronutrients** that are carbohydrates, fats, proteins, and water.

Carbohydrates

You need carbohydrates, also known as carbs, to give your body its primary source of energy. If you have ever tried to severely restrict your carb intake, you know that your level of functioning decreases and so does your overall feeling of wellness. In fact, restricting carbs below the recommended daily amount will leave you weak in the knees, fatigued, and feeling like howling at the moon. Carbs from whole unrefined foods give you the energy you need and supply vitamins, minerals, and fiber for proper cell and organ function.

def•i•ni•tion

Carbs are grouped into two main categories **complex** (starches) or **simple** (sugars), depending on how fast your body digests and absorbs the sugar. The more complex, the longer it takes to digest.

Complex carbs give your body a slow, steady energy supply because they are absorbed and metabolized slowly. *Simple carbs* are easily digested and absorbed so they increase blood sugar supplies quickly, often exceeding cell requirements for energy and ending up being stored as fat.

Eating a continual oversupply of simple carbs from table and refined sugar, cookies, soda, and refined and processed foods might take you down the road to having metabolic problems such as type 2 or adult onset diabetes. But on the flip side, if you don't get the required minimum amount of carbohydrates, your body begins to break down fat for energy, causing by-products called ketone bodies to build up in the blood and altering normal pH balance. Although this might sound great if you want to lose weight, altering normal pH balance is not healthy and a continual state of acidosis at the very basic level impairs your body's ability to function and heal itself.

In other words, there's no way around it—you need to get 40 to 65 percent of your calories (depending on activity level) from a variety of unprocessed and unrefined carbohydrate-based foods such as fruits, vegetables, whole grains, whole wheat bread, brown rice, whole-grain pasta, peas, beans, and whole oats. And, yes, fruit has simple carbs, but it also has fiber and other vital nutrients that work synergistically to fuel, nourish, and support your body. Fiber also helps to slow the digestive process, which in turn slows down the rate of sugar absorbed into your bloodstream.

Proteins

Most of your body is made of protein and maintained with a regular protein intake. Proteins (amino acids) are either essential or nonessential. Your body needs about 13 nonessential amino acids (proteins that don't have to come from your diet because your body can make them) and 9 essential amino acids (proteins that cannot be made in your body but must come from the food you eat).

Some foods are complete protein sources because they supply enough essential amino acids; others are incomplete protein because they don't supply all the essential amino acids. All meat and other animal products, including beef, lamb, pork, poultry, fish, shellfish, eggs, milk, and milk products are complete protein foods. Grains, fruits, and vegetables are low, incomplete, or lack one of the essential amino acids and are considered incomplete protein foods.

People on vegetarian diets should combine proteins so they include all the essential amino acids to form a complete protein. For example, you can combine rice and beans, milk and wheat cereal, or corn and beans to make a complete protein meal. Most adults need two to three servings of protein-rich food daily to maintain health.

Fats

Fats give you a concentrated source of energy, provide the building blocks for cell membranes, are necessary to incorporate calcium into bones, protect the heart and liver, enhance the immune system, protect against harmful organisms in the GI tract, and are essential for the synthesis of hormones and other substances.

Fat in your diet makes you feel satisfied after a meal and keeps you from overeating. It supplies vital fat-soluble vitamins A, D, E, and K and is necessary to convert carotene in food to vitamin A for mineral absorption and many other body processes and functions.

Essential fatty acids (EFAs) omega-3 and omega-6 must be obtained through diet. Omega-9 is a nonessential fatty acid because the body can make it from essential EFAs you consume. Essential fatty acids raise your good cholesterol, called HDL, which takes the bad cholesterol (LDL) to the liver to be broken down and excreted.

Energy Bar

According to recent research, 1 gram of an omega-3 fatty acid a day from sources like cod liver oil can decrease symptoms of depression such as anxiety, sadness, and sleeping problems after twelve weeks of use.

The omega-6 fatty acid is used by your body to make hormones and to increase inflammation (an important part of the immune response), as well as for blood clotting and cell production. Most processed foods have high levels of omega-6s so it's overly prevalent in the American diet. Omega-6 comes from seeds, nuts, and oils—particularly vegetable oils. Our bodies need the inflammatory response for immune function, but the imbalance that's been caused by overprevalence of omega-6 in the American diet is thought to be partly the cause of the rise in inflammatory and autoimmune diseases such as heart disease, arthritis, and cancer. The omega-3 fatty acids eicosapentaenoic (EPA) and docosa-hexaenoic (DHA) are critical for synthesis of hormones that control immune function and work to boost immune system function by increasing the activity of white blood cells that consume bacteria (phagocytes). They protect against damage and the stress response of infections, play a part in blood clotting, and are building blocks for cells and cell membranes.

Many studies have shown that getting the recommended amounts of DHA and EPA by eating fish (or taking fish oil supplements) has the following health effects:

◆ Lowers triglyceride levels and reduces your risk of death, heart attack, sometimes fatal abnormal heart rhythms, and strokes and slows the buildup of atherosclerotic plaques that cause hardening of the arteries.

◆ Reduces the risk of blood clots that can cause strokes, heart attacks, deep vein thrombosis, and embolisms in the lungs.

◆ Lowers blood pressure.

◆ Prevents or reduces symptoms of inflammatory diseases including arthritis, migraine headaches, menstrual cramps, and asthma. Reducing inflammation also reduces pain that contributes to fatigue.

◆ Protects vision.

◆ Protects against depression and other mood disorders and improves concentration. Mood disorders are often linked to fatigue.

◆ Reduces the risk of cancer and strengthens the immune system. CFS and stress-related conditions are linked in part to weakened immune system function.

◆ Reduces risk of osteoporosis by playing a part in rebuilding bone.

Omega-3s are scarce in the American diet and are found mostly in the fat of cold-water fish such as salmon, sardines, mackerel, black cod, herring, and bluefish. You can also get omega-3 in some grains (wheat) and nuts (walnuts), eggs, organ meats, fish, and green vegetables if the meats, fish, and plants are raised naturally and organically.

The ratio of omega-6 to omega-3 fats is ideally 1:1, but today the more common ratio is 20:1 or higher. You can get a balance of the right kinds of fats by eating a variety of lean meat from grass-fed animals, organic butter, fruits, vegetables, grains, oily fish, extra virgin olive oil, sesame seed oil, grape seed oil, unrefined flax seed oil in small amounts, coconut oil, and egg yolks. Or by eating 5 ounces of nuts and 12 ounces of mercury- and PCB-free fish like Atlantic or Alaskan salmon, mahi-mahi, tilapia, freshwater bass, catfish, flounder, sole, herring, and whitefish every week, you will get the right amount of EFAs. EFAs are destroyed by light, air, and heat, so buy cold- or expeller-pressed oils in opaque glass containers and store them in the refrigerator after opening.

Water

Your body is about two-thirds water, or 40 to 50 quarts, and your brain is about 70 percent water. You need water to digest nutrients, for every body function and process, to stay lubricated and cooled, to dispose of waste, and to fight disease. Dehydration is a common reason to feel fatigued, tired, or sluggish.

Some people tend to feel hungry all the time, which could be due to chronic dehydration. Make sure you are adequately hydrated all day by drinking plenty of water. Divide your body weight in half and drink that many ounces of water a day if you are sedentary. For active people, use 75 percent of your body weight as a guide.

In The Know

"By not drinking enough water, many people incur excess body fat, poor muscle tone and size, decreased digestive efficiency and organ function, increased toxicity in the body, joint and muscle soreness, and water retention."

—Dr. Howard Flaks, obesity specialist, Beverly Hills, California

---

Vitamins and Minerals

Unlike carbohydrates, protein, and fats, vitamins don't provide energy when they are broken down. So, those vitamin or mineral waters and energy bars that claim to give you a pick-me-up are simply untrue marketing ploys. You do, however, need micronutrients to prevent disease, to stay healthy, and for proper body functions.

There are 13 vitamins necessary for health: vitamins A, C, D, E, K, and the B vitamins (thiamine, riboflavin, niacin, pantothenic acid, biotin, vitamin B_6, vitamin B_{12}, and folate). All except D and K need to come from the foods you eat; vitamins D and K can be synthesized in the body.

A balanced diet of a variety of real whole foods is your best way to get the vital nutrients and phytochemicals you need for peak immune function. But a deficiency in just a single nutrient from a less-than-optimal diet can overwhelm your immune function. The shining stars of immune function protective nutrients are the antioxidants, especially vitamins C and E, beta-carotene, and the mineral zinc. Phytochemicals are non-nutritive plant chemicals with protective, disease preventive properties that come in sufficient quantities from eating your five to nine servings of fruits and vegetables everyday.

Get Your C

Vitamin C or ascorbic acid is a *water-soluble* vitamin that must be obtained through diet because it can't be synthesized in the body. You need vitamin C to make collagen, a structural component of tendons, ligaments, blood vessels, and bone. You also need vitamin C to synthesize the neurotransmitter norepinephrine that is critical for certain brain functions and healthy mood. Your body needs vitamin C for the processes that result in cellular energy and to metabolize cholesterol to bile acids, which in turn affects blood cholesterol levels and might lower the incidence of gallstones.

Vitamin C is a powerful antioxidant that has major immune-boosting effects and is used in the production of infection-fighting white blood cells and antibodies. It increases your body's level of interferon, which is your natural defense against viral infections including colds and flu, and has its own interferon-like properties. Vitamin C is also known to reduce your risk of cardiovascular disease by raising HDL (good) cholesterol levels and lowering blood pressure, and it helps to reduce plaque in the arteries. Diets higher in vitamin C have also proven to lower rates of colon, prostate, and breast cancer.

Great food sources of vitamin C are asparagus, celery, pineapples, lettuce, watermelon, fennel, broccoli, bell peppers, kale, cauliflower, strawberries, kiwi, snow peas, cantaloupe, oranges, grapefruit, limes, lemons, mustard and turnip greens, brussels sprouts, papaya, chard, cabbage, spinach, tomatoes, zucchini, raspberries, peppermint, and parsley.

E Is for Elementary

Vitamin E is a fat-soluble vitamin and is another important and powerful antioxidant vital for healthy immune system function. Vitamin E stimulates the production of natural killer cells whose function is to seek and destroy illness-causing organisms and other invaders such as cancer cells. It also enhances the production of certain immune cells or B-cells whose function is to produce antibodies to destroy bacteria. Vitamin E is thought to lower the risk of cardiovascular disease, including heart attacks. It is found in seeds and grains.

Beta What?

Beta-carotene is the third major antioxidant that works against free radicals and enhances immune system function by increasing natural killer cells and helper T-cells (infection-fighting cells). Studies show it also helps to reduce the risk of cardiovascular disease by interfering with the production of arterial plaque. It also stimulates macrophages (immune cells) to produce tumor necrosis factor that destroys cancer cells.

Beta-carotene is a member of the carotenoid family that works synergistically with all the other carotenoids found in a real whole food healthy diet for optimal immune function.

Beta-carotene is converted to vitamin A (a fat-soluble vitamin) in the body, another anticancer and immune-boosting vitamin. Your body stops making vitamin A when it has enough, and too much vitamin A is toxic to the body which is why you should get necessary carotene from foods.

Rounding Out the Vitamin Alphabet

Zinc is a mineral that increases the production and boosts the activity of infection-fighting white blood cells. Zinc has anticancer properties and increases the number of T-cells. It is found in oysters, crab, beef, turkey, and beans.

It Isn't Just About Flavor

Bioflavenoids are a group of phytonutrients that assist the immune system by protecting against environmental pollutants. They also lessen the production of plaque from cholesterol and reduce the formation of microscopic clots within arteries that often lead to heart attack and stroke. Eat at least six servings per day of a wide variety of fruits and vegetables to get the bioflavenoids you need.

Selenium is another mineral that increases natural killer cells and activates cancer-fighting cells. You can get the selenium you need from tuna, brown rice, egg yolks, cottage cheese, chicken (white meat), red snapper, lobster, shrimp, whole grains, organic vegetables, sunflower seeds, garlic, Brazil nuts, and lamb chops.

What Is Real Food?

Real food can be identified as something that was growing and alive at one time, that spoils, that usually requires some sort of preparation, that has flavor specific to its species, and that has varied colors and textures specific to its type. A diet of real whole food consists of meals and snacks that are prepared using produce, dairy, meat, fish, nuts, whole grains, oils, legumes, and seeds.

Aside from nourishing your body and keeping you healthy, real food has an added benefit of not being fattening. While processed, junk, and convenience foods have a strong link to obesity and degenerative diseases, there is little to no correlation between a diet that consists of a wide variety of real whole food in the proper ratio of fat, protein, and carbohydrates to obesity or disease.

Jessica is a 30-year-old mother of two boys that she homeschools. Three years ago she was overweight, depressed, fatigued, and plagued with headaches, body aches, and allergies. She was only 27 years old, but she felt 60!

Jessica decided that what she'd heard about the importance of nutrition might just be the ticket out of feeling sick and fat and prematurely old. She did a drastic turn around of her and her family's diet by eliminating processed junk foods and soda. She started to exercise regularly and without actually dieting immediately began to lose weight and to feel more energized. Her chronic headaches and pain also improved along with her overall mood.

Jessica loves to bake, but she found that by using wholesome ingredients like whole wheat flour, real cocoa, and sucanant (dried sugar cane), she can still serve her family great deserts without processed ingredients. Three years later she's 40 pounds lighter, she feels great and even her kids are better behaved. While you might not be able to make the immediate changes Jessica did, you can implement slow changes that will give you similar results.

Managing Low Blood Sugar

When you eat sugar, or something that can be converted quickly into sugar in your body, your blood sugar rises quickly with a corresponding rise in insulin to keep your blood sugar steady. This then causes your blood sugar to drop too low too quickly, causing symptoms of low blood sugar, or *hypoglycemia*. In other words, eating sugar causes hypoglycemia. And the main symptom of hypoglycemia is fatigue, which makes managing symptoms of hypoglycemia crucial in winning your fight against fatigue.

Many people are lured into eating sugar for the temporary quick fix of energy it provides. But in people with hypoglycemia, the continual quick sugar fix only makes the condition worsen over time. The first step in your management of hypoglycemia is to avoid sugar and simple carbs in your diet. Simple carbs include table sugar, corn syrup, bread and pasta made with white flour, bakery goods made with white flour, soda, fruit juice, candy, cake, ice cream, and most packaged cereal.

Another way to avoid sugar is to stay away from processed and packaged foods. They are generally high sugar in the form of corn syrup, corn sweetener, and high fructose corn syrup. Even processed lunch meats and such seemingly innocent foods as ketchup contain hidden sugar ingredients such as high fructose corn syrup.

Something else to stay away from is caffeine because caffeine stimulates the release of blood glucose, which is one reason caffeine helps you feel awake and gives you a false sense of energy. If you tend to use caffeine for a crutch to keep your energy levels up, then you probably are putting yourself in a cycle of peaks and valleys that will tend to worsen over time and you should quit or reduce caffeine. If you cannot go without your morning cup of coffee, at least avoid putting sugar in it and try adding some fresh organic milk or cream to provide some good nutrients and balance.

 Slip-Ups

To avoid hypoglycemia, never skip meals or go longer than two to three hours without a nonsugar snack or meal. Sugar, white flour, alcohol, caffeine, and tobacco all cause or worsen low blood sugar and should be limited or avoided entirely.

Begin your program of balancing your blood sugar with three well-balanced meals, starting with a good and balanced breakfast, and three in-between meal snacks. If you still have symptoms, you might need to decrease your meal size and increase the number of times you eat. Smaller, more frequent meals help to release glucose into your bloodstream more gradually and evenly.

As you plan your meals, make sure that you stick with complex carbs such as whole-grain pasta, fresh vegetables and fruits, whole grains, beans, peas, oats, and brown rice because they take longer to break down in your intestine and help to keep blood glucose levels more level.

Proteins and fats also take longer to be absorbed and converted into glucose by the body. Ideally, eat fruits whole along with a fat and protein. For example, an apple with cheese will keep your blood sugar steadier than an apple alone and you will also be getting your portion of fat.

As you move toward eating a healthy diet, start a food diary. Write down everything you consume over the course of a week or two, including food, drink, and medications you take as well as the time at which you consume it. Also, record any symptoms you experience and the time they begin. After a couple of days, you might begin to see a correlation between what you take in and the symptoms it causes. As you recognize this cause and effect, you can begin to take steps to eliminate those things that have an adverse affect on your health. One word of warning, though. If it is your medication that is causing some of your symptoms, do not stop taking it. Instead, please discuss your situation with your doctor.

When to Eat

We've discussed a bit about what to eat; now we probably should talk about *when* you should eat. Let's start by what not to do.

One cause of fatigue is often the result of the crash, jolt, crash cycle of eating. You skip breakfast, eat a salad for lunch, and feel a crash coming on around 2 P.M. To jump-start your energy, you grab some caffeine or a sugary snack and jolt your system awake. After a while, you begin to drift off again, and feeling the crash coming on, head back to the vending machine for another jolt. Habits like skipping meals, binging, and not eating breakfast end up giving your body mixed signals that can lead to feelings of continual hunger and fatigue.

Although there are many theories about the number of meals to eat, how often, and when to eat, those who don't have problems with hypoglycemia typically need only three meals a day with healthy snacks in between. The most basic premise is to eat when you really feel hungry but don't wait until you feel starved. It's generally accepted that you if eat at regular intervals, your body's metabolism will not be negatively affected and you won't tend to store extra calories in the form of fat. Of course, this implies that you are eating whole healthy food in the proper ratio of protein, fats, and carbohydrates.

Energy Bar

Plan meals so that you are getting 6 to 11 servings of whole grains, 2 to 4 servings of fruit, 3 to 5 servings of vegetables, and 3 cups of quality dairy products every day.

If you feel better eating small frequent meals, that's the route you should take. But no matter how many meals you eat each day, be sure that the quality of what you are eating and the number of calories are balanced by your activity level.

The following basic tips will help you determine a schedule of eating that will best suit you:

◆ Make breakfast a priority. You need to start your day with enough fuel for your body to function optimally and so that your metabolism doesn't shut down and cause you to store fat more easily when you do eat.

◆ Eat meals at regular scheduled times, three to four hours apart.

◆ When you feel hungry in between meals, have some herbal tea or water and wait another twenty minutes to see if you still feel hungry.

◆ Snacks help keep your metabolism at an even keel and prevent binging. Eat a nutritious snack in between meals. The fiber, fat, protein, and carbohydrate from whole foods will help keep your blood sugar level and your brain happy and satisfied between meals.

◆ Eat your last full meal no later than two to three hours before bed. Eating right before bed can keep you awake by causing GI distress or by causing your body to work on metabolizing the food when that time is needed by your body to rest. It also might cause you to not feel hungry in the morning so that you don't eat your necessary breakfast.

Tips for Eating Right

If you do not have the best of eating habits right now, all the information in this chapter might seem daunting. It is a lot to process, especially if you do not have a lot of energy. However, making some simple changes will go a long way to improving your diet. To begin with, taking the time to plan out your meals is key to a healthy diet. Planning ahead allows you to make sure you have the food you need on hand, when you need it. It also makes that trip to the grocery store a little less stressful because you know exactly what you need to buy rather than wandering aimlessly through the store, buying processed foods because they will be "quick and easy" to prepare. Remember, too, when you are grocery shopping that if you don't have unhealthy foods in your pantry you are less likely to eat something you will regret in times of weakness.

As you are planning your meals and grocery list, think about shopping in the periphery of the supermarket where the produce and meats are and look for labels that say organic or, in the case of meats, raised without hormones or antibiotics. Organic is better quality and is toxin free. If you can't buy organic produce, wash your produce in a tub of water with a cup of vinegar to remove any traces of pesticides.

After you've returned from the store, take some time to work ahead. If you can take some time to do some meal preparation ahead of time, make a meal and freeze it, or at least know what you are going to have for the next meal, you might be less likely to give in to the temptation of going out to eat or getting take-out. Your meal probably will be healthier, too.

Start on your new healthy food diet by making changes gradually. The worst thing you can do is to go from a typical American diet of junk and processed food to trying to eat a diet of wheat grass and bean sprouts because you will end up feeling defeated and most likely give up. Besides, a healthy diet isn't extreme—it's a balance of real whole foods such as lean meats and poultry, whole grains and brown rice, beans, produce, healthy oils such as extra virgin olive oil, nuts, seeds, and dairy. Use a small amount of oil for cooking meats and sautéing because you want to cook only the food, not the oil. If you eat a lot of processed and fast food, try replacing one of those meals a week with a whole food meal you prepare yourself and add whole food snacks.

Begin your new adventure into preparing healthy food by preparing very basic meals such as grilled or roasted meat and chicken. Serve the meat with whole-wheat rolls with butter and a salad or vegetables. Instead of rolls for complex carbohydrates, try some whole-grain pasta with a vegetable-based or low-fat sauce.

Salad is another healthy, simple meal to prepare. Salad can be made with almost any vegetable and can be a hearty meal if you add some grilled meat, chicken, fish, or cheese and eat it with whole-grain bread and butter. Be careful, though. The worst thing you can do to salad is to pour on it bottled salad dressing that is chock full of chemicals. Be sure if you do buy prepared dressing that it's organic with ingredients that you can recognize. Better yet, make your own dressing using vinegar and extra virgin olive oil in a ratio of 1:2 with a bit of honey and Dijon mustard, salt, and pepper. Depending on what kind of oil and vinegar you use, the taste of your dressing will vary.

Here are a few more simple tips to get you eating better. Buy a blender and a food processor because both will cut your meal preparation time and make cooking easier. Get some large cooking pots so you can make bigger quantities of soups and sauces to freeze. A thermos is a great way to bring a hot lunch to work. You can take leftovers from the night before, cut up some fruits and vegetables, and put some nuts and pieces of cheese and crackers in a sandwich bag for quick and easy meals at work. Remember to look for crackers that are chemical free and made without oils.

In The Know
"The reason we are so tired begins with the Standard American Diet, which features 150 pounds of sugar a year, white flour, and almost no fiber. It's dreadful! This is the first time in the history of the world that we have high-calorie malnutrition." —Jacob Teitelbaum, M.D., *author of* From Fatigued to Fantastic

Use garlic as often as possible because it is a powerful immune system booster. It enhances the multiplication of white cells, boosts natural killer cell action, amplifies efficiency of antibody production, and acts as an antioxidant by reducing free radicals in the bloodstream.

Stay away from grocery store salt. Instead, use sea salt. Sea salt is essential for tasty meal preparation and gives you the sodium you need in your diet in a healthy way.

When you switch from eating processed to real whole food, your taste buds will change over time and you will begin to enjoy real food more and stop craving food that's not good for you. The best motivation to eat right will come after you begin to feel better, have more energy, and most likely lose weight in a very short time.

The Least You Need to Know

- Eat a balanced diet of real whole food in a ratio of about 40 percent carbohydrates, 30 percent protein, and 30 percent fat for health and healing your fatigue state.

- Real food was alive or growing at one time and doesn't contain components injurious to health such as additives and preservatives.

- Manage symptoms of blood sugar by eating frequent, small, well-balanced meals and snacks and avoid sugar, caffeine, neurotoxins, and smoking.

- Most people need to eat only three meals a day about three to four hours apart with snacks in between, starting with a good breakfast. Never skip meals.

- Make dietary changes gradually by substituting one processed or junk food meal a week with a meal prepared with real whole food and by eating whole-food snacks. Motivation follows changes in diet from improvements in your health.

Exercise and Daily Activity

In This Chapter

- ◆ Accepting your limitations
- ◆ Dealing with post exertional malaise
- ◆ The importance of pacing
- ◆ The basics of graded exercise
- ◆ Keeping it real
- ◆ How naps and rest help

Depending on the severity, your fatigue might force you to make some dramatic changes in your lifestyle. You may need to decrease or even eliminate some of your usual activities, and how you deal with this can in fact impact the course of your recovery.

You might find for the first time in your life that you need to limit your work, your play, and your life in general, but the truth is fatigue requires a different approach to activity and exercise, including planning and setting limits. The good news is if you do this limit-setting correctly, early on, and intelligently, then it can not only get you back into the game sooner, but can also prevent you from suffering with increased and even debilitating fatigue.

Twenty years ago when illnesses such as Chronic Fatigue Syndrome (CFS) were first emerging, people were told that their condition didn't exist. They were losing their jobs and their lifestyles without even the support of their doctors, much less employers and friends. These people suffered without validation and didn't have much hope of recovery. Consider, though, that these days we have the benefit of having information at hand and you also have the reassurance that by taking the right steps, making the right changes, and giving yourself hope you can and will recover.

Whether you have mild or severe fatigue, the principles for recovery are the same. This chapter will help you understand some of what you have been experiencing in regard to activity, exercise, and fatigue and how to deal with it. You also will learn how to set up a program of exercise and why it's important—and even vital—to your recovery from fatigue.

Understanding Limitations

The hardest thing to do when you become fatigued, ill, or faced with making changes is to accept new limitations in your life. The fact is that you cannot go on like you used to and you need to step back, reorder your life, and (depending on your level of fatigue) slow down and begin to say no. Slowing down can take a lot of acceptance on your part, including understanding and accepting how some excessive behavior factors into your fatigue. For example, if you are a person who has exercised to excess, finding yourself in a state of forced slowdown most likely is very difficult to accept, and very difficult to understand.

Setting limits can include reducing your working hours or even completely stopping work, even if it is only until you recover. If your identity is strongly tied to your work or to exercise or another activity, then accepting your limitations will be even more difficult and painful. But it's a vital part of your recovery, and you must look at it as part of your healing process and as a door that is closing while another one opens.

By learning and accepting information, you will be able to keep yourself on track without feeding any toxic negativity. Fatigue might have brought you to your knees, but it is so you can stop and reevaluate the many aspects of your life that brought you there. Understanding your current limitations will help you to accept and embrace the other changes that need to take place.

Exercise Intolerance

Perhaps you've been a very busy overextended person, you're used to days that are filled with multitasking, or you have many responsibilities. Maybe fatigue has brought you to a quiet and still place that you might not identify with, so you take advantage of those days you have more energy to do the things you're dying to do. But then it seems, out of nowhere, that you are hit with fatigue that is even worse. What's the deal? You are pushing past your limits without knowing it. The crash and burn you experience after participating in a seemingly innocent activity is known as *exercise intolerance* or *post exertional malaise (PEM)*.

Another chapter used a savings account as an analogy to good health. So fatigue, depending on the severity, can be compared to continually withdrawing money from your account without making many deposits. You simply have exceeded your energy stores or savings account, and you might have been living on borrowed energy, running on empty, or using false energy-like stimulants. When you reach a state of severe fatigue, you won't be able to get energy from any source—even the loan sharks such as caffeine—and any activity will cause you to have PEM.

def•i•ni•tion

Post exertional malaise (PEM) is a hallmark of certain fatigue states and a diagnostic marker for CFS. It is defined by a worsening of fatigue and related symptoms for a period of at least twenty-four hours after exertion, activity, or exercise.

While researchers still aren't sure why those with CFS don't tolerate aerobic exercise (or even activities of daily living like hygiene and dressing), there are several theories including:

◆ Mitochondria are the energy factories within the cells, and a disruption in their ability to function causes an inability to generate energy with aerobic or any other activity.

◆ There are defects in cellular respiration, which is the process where chemical bonds of molecules including glucose are converted into energy to be used by the cells.

◆ There is a dysregulation of the autonomic nervous system and hypothalamic-pituitary-adrenal axis limiting the body's ability to deal with stress, including physical stress.

◆ You might have a chronic infection or an activation of a dormant infection.

◆ You have a dysregulated immune or inflammatory system.

Energy Bar

People with fatigue have to deal with activity in a different way than healthy people do. For that reason, you need learn to say no and to explain to others that contrary to their suggestions, you won't feel better if you just get out.

In other words, your vital systems that are supposed to finely modulate your hormones and back you up during times of stress are so hammered that they are no longer able to do their jobs. You are not generating energy to your cells, and your ability to recover also is compromised.

PEM typically lasts at least twenty-four hours, but for some people it lasts much longer. It's very defeating to exceed your limitations and experience PEM. Continue reading to learn how to realize your limitations; stay within your boundaries; slowly heal; and build back your strength, reserves, and endurance.

What Is Pacing?

Pacing is a strategy in fatigue recovery based on building strength and endurance while preventing PEM. It's a method that's useful for anyone regardless of whether they have mild or severe fatigue. Pacing refers to the continual planning for rest, expending energy only within your limitations, stopping before you have any symptoms, and gradually increasing energy expenditure only when you have enough saved. The aim is to remain active but to not overdo and suffer the crash and burn. This might seem like common sense, but it's human nature to be active and act "well" when you are feeling better. But it's confusing and defeating when you suffer the consequences without knowing why. Pacing requires a continual evaluation and reevaluation of your energy savings and level of endurance and pulling back as necessary to get needed rest.

Pacing is a way of managing your lifestyle depending on the here and now. It requires that you listen to your body. If you have the energy, you can engage in or continue an activity, but you stop before you are tired—and certainly when you feel any symptoms, you stop. Pacing also requires that you assess your level of energy savings before you start something and say no to things that you can't do without exceeding your savings. The great thing about pacing is that when done right and with discipline, it really works.

Now that you understand PEM, perhaps you can factor that into a clearer understanding of your bad days and stop beating yourself up. Because it's our nature to want to be well, and be well *now*, it's easy to overdo and extend our energy on days when we feel better. That's the downside of pacing. It's very hard to have the discipline you need to say no, to pull back, and to stop before you are tired.

In The Know

"The vast majority of patients I see get well with my standard work up with respect to a) vitamins and minerals, b) diet, c) pacing, and d) sleep. All these things must be put in place to repair and prevent ongoing damage to mitochondria so allowing them to recover. For mitochondria to recover they need all the essential vitamins, minerals, essential fatty acids and amino acids to manufacture the cellular machinery to restore normal function."

—*Dr. Sarah Myhill, United Kingdom physician and pioneer in the treatment of CFS*

The fact is that in fatigue recovery, "just because you can doesn't mean that you should." In fact, to really build endurance it's absolutely mandatory to pace by doing only half of what you feel you can do. For example, if you feel like cleaning your house, only clean one or two rooms. If you want to exercise, only do half of that yoga class or DVD. It takes some discipline, some disappointments, and some practice at assessing your level of energy and fatigue to do this.

Pacing doesn't include setting goals; instead you increase your activity only when you can. And because it can include setbacks, you cannot feed yourself any sort of negativity with internal dialogue that you are a loser or "not yourself," because you aren't going full speed. Take on a mindset of being accepting and good to yourself.

How Pacing Factors into Recovery

If you do not cut your energy expenditure in half, you can experience PEM beginning either later that day or when you wake up the next day. PEM is not fun, is often painful, is demoralizing and defeating, and only causes you to fall further behind in your recovery. It doesn't take very long to figure out what will cause you to experience PEM. And once you do, simply ratchet down the amount of energy you spend on your next good day.

The flip side of saving half of your energy is that you can add it to your energy bank account, increasing its value. The time you spend resting is actually working to heal your body. Whereas the time you are forced to rest during times of PEM is not really being invested in your healing—it's just being used to recover from the overexertion. By pacing your energy expenditure over time, you will be able to slowly build up your reserves and endurance and be able to increase your activity level.

Remember, if you feel better on any given day, don't be tempted to do too much or you will cause more damage and further postpone your recovery. Healthy pacing requires that you feel well without any symptoms during times of rest and inactivity before you increase your level of activity. You can't force your recovery. It's not a mind over matter issue—it's an issue of physiological and biochemical restoration that needs all the components of healing, diet, rest, and exercise with a balanced approach to progress and heal.

Pacing Requirements

Your pacing requirements will depend on your level of fatigue. Some people such as those with CFS, those recovering from chemotherapy, or those with multiple sclerosis (MS) can have such severe fatigue that something as seemingly innocuous as talking will cause PEM. So setting your requirements may take looking at your daily activities, figuring out what you must do versus what is optional, and then bargaining down even further. Remember that your goal is having your energy bank account in the black again and that you have to save, save, save to make that happen.

It can help to first factor in more rest than activity and slowly add a little exertion on good days to "test the waters." If that works, then increase but pull back immediately with any symptoms of weariness, low energy, pain, or muscle weakness. Also watch for other symptoms, including GI symptoms or allergy symptoms, because any physical symptom is a red flag for a run-in with PEM.

Energy Bar _____

Even though you plan ahead, you always have to be ready to pull back. Try to balance enjoyable activities and work in the same day and stop to rest before you feel any symptoms.

Another critical aspect of pacing is to not do too little or to rest too much. You might be groaning or even saying, "Come on!" But the truth is it's a very fine balancing act that you have to do continually because too much activity will cause PEM, but too little will cause deconditioning. That can be just another hurdle that you have to overcome because it will drag you down further. Writing down your goals for activity can help you to stay within them and meet them at the same time. If you are able to consistently do one activity without suffering with PEM, you should keep that activity as a regular and work in others.

Realistic Exercise

A healthy person feels invigorated during and after exercise, even vigorous grueling exercise. However, a person with fatigue must exercise within his tolerable limits and often has low endurance and little strength, becomes tired easily, and might experience PEM. Realistic exercise for you then is anything you are able to do without becoming tired while you are doing it or suffering later with PEM.

The first thing to do in planning your exercise is to keep in mind that your tolerance is going to vary from day to day. That's why it's a good idea to keep a diary of exercise goals along with outcomes. That way, you can see that you did some chores or walked for twenty minutes and didn't suffer a relapse. Then after a few weeks, you can try to increase your time by five minutes. If that doesn't work, then pull back. Don't forget to factor in other activities because it might not have been the extra five minutes of walking that did you in. Your PEM might be due to some other energy expenditure that day.

The truth is that exercise can mean one thing to you and something else to another person. If you are moving your body, you are exercising, and moving is critically important to prevent deconditioning. If you have severe fatigue, then any activity where you move your body or lift any weight "counts" as your exercise.

Graded Exercise

Without exercise, your body grows weaker, your muscles further atrophy, and you become less able to defend against illness and increasing fatigue. Fatigue takes the element of feeling in control away, but by exercising and reconditioning, you can start to regain control of your life.

PEM causes a circle of avoidance due to its Pavlovian-type conditioning of correlating exercise and activity with punishment. But not exercising leads to deconditioning, which only makes any activity harder so that you begin experiencing PEM with milder activities like the ordinary activities of daily living. For this reason, you have to approach exercise in the slow, methodic systematic way that is known as *graded exercise*.

def•i•ni•tion

Graded exercise is a planned exercise program that starts out slowly and increases in very small steps. This means you stay within your plan even on good days when you feel like doing more. By staying within your plan, you are less likely to exceed your energy savings while you build strength and endurance.

The difference between pacing and graded exercise is that with pacing you don't plan ahead and set goals because you use the here and now to set your level of activity. Graded exercise, however, requires a methodical plan that you stick with, you don't exceed even when you feel you can, and you increase in small energy expending increments as you are able to.

Planning Your Workout

Healthy people can jump out of bed, exercise, and then get on with their day. But people with fatigue who exercise early in the day will use up their allotted energy more quickly and might find that they become overly tired and even experience PEM. So plan your exercise for after lunch or even later in the day because it's more easily tolerated and has an added bonus of helping with sleep. Just be sure you don't exercise in the three to four hours before going to bed because you need those hours to wind down.

It's a good idea to work in about three exercise sessions a week, beginning your program with stretching such as gentle yoga and alternating with other types like Tai Chi. Because these early sessions are designed to not be strenuous, you also can take advantage of the time to do deep-breathing techniques, pray, and meditate at the same time.

When you become stronger, gradually move from stretching to strengthening activities using very light weights. You can use some light stretch bands or even just your body weight. Start with a session of just one half-minute of lifting weights, pulling the bands, or lifting and lowering your arms or legs and then several minutes of rest. Repeat this up to five times. Work up your time slowly by increasing your time and weights only after several weeks. When you are tolerating the session, gradually increase your sessions to two a day, then three a day, and so on. In the beginning, breaking your sessions into single five-minute blocks—three five-minute sessions a day will be better tolerated than one fifteen-minute session if you have severe fatigue with PEM.

After you have done some conditioning with stretching and low weights and are able to tolerate it without any relapse, you can start some aerobic exercise. Begin by walking only a very short distance in short time frames (say, five minutes) and increase your time and distance only when you can tolerate it without becoming tired and with zero symptoms of PEM the following day.

Don't forget to factor in all your activity. If you have been relatively active during the day, it might not be a good day for you to walk. Aerobic activity is the most difficult to do without relapse if your fatigue is severe.

For all exercise, allow recovery days in between. Factor in all other stressors so that you are not overdoing it. If you can, use a heart rate monitor to keep tabs on your heart rate during exercise, or simply take your pulse. Until you reach a point of conditioning where you are not experiencing any PEM, you should not exceed 90 to 110 beats per minute. A normal heart rate is 60 to 100 beats per minute, depending on factors such as age and conditioning. Exercise target heart rate ranges are typically calculated using percentages. If you have severe fatigue or CFS you also have decreased exercise capacity, so keeping an eye on your heart rate is going to help you avoid PEM.

Because some people with severe fatigue also have problems with autonomic dysfunction, they sometimes experience orthostatic intolerance (OI). A person with OI doesn't compensate with normal blood pressure and heart rate when standing; rather she has an increase in heart rate and a decrease in blood pressure that causes symptoms including fatigue, tremors, breathing or swallowing difficulties, headache, visual disturbances, light-headedness, dizziness, nausea, sweating, and pallor. If you have any of these symptoms when exercising, make sure you see a doctor to get cleared for any exercise program. Your doctor may want to rule out other serious health issues before giving you a diagnosis of autonomic dysfunction.

If you have OI, you need to do your exercises lying down or sitting in cool water (hot water causes the blood vessels to dilate and thus increases your OI symptoms). Try volume loading with fluid prior to any standing or any other upright activity. Seriously, by chugging down an eight-ounce bottle of

> **Slip-Ups**
>
> Don't be tempted by a sudden surge of energy to do something that exceeds your energy savings. Remember: you have to stay within your graded exercise plan to make consistent gains and to avoid suffering the negative consequences of PEM.

water you can raise your blood pressure within fifteen minutes and sustain that pressure for up to an hour.

Finally, be consistent but cautious and aware of your body so that you can pace in a healthy way, recondition your body with your graded exercise plan, and have few or no setbacks.

Recognizing Your Limits

The time you are in recovery from fatigue often feels like being on the bench while the rest of the team is having a great time playing. Even though you might want to slip into feeling sorry for yourself, you have to realize that there is a season for all things and your convalescence so to speak is your season to heal.

Part of that realization is first becoming aware, then accepting, and then staying within your limits in all your activities—not just exercise. Because staying within your limits is so important for fatigue recovery, the first essential step is to do away with any guilt, self-pity, or low self-esteem that might be caused by your inability to deal with and engage in "normal" things and life.

Staying within your limits also means telling others that you cannot do certain activities (or be around certain thing such as fragrances) without being apologetic. Although some people will never understand, others will and the bottom line is that exceeding your limits for the sake of not offending someone or not embarrassing yourself is only going to hurt you, cause more damage, and slow your recovery.

Keeping your written record can help you to see the amount of time and the types of activities you can do during the course of a day without experiencing PEM or other symptoms. You can then list activities that have minimal or no risk, those with moderate risk, and those that are absolutely "no can do" activities.

Energy Bar

You can extend your energy levels by "switching" or changing activities so that you avoid tiring muscle groups. For example, if you have been working on the computer, you are straining your eye muscles and back muscles. Getting up to do a different activity can help you stay active without becoming fatigued.

Activities don't have to be physical to cause symptoms. Reading; using a computer; and emotional states like worry, anger, arguing, and depression also can worsen fatigue. Keeping an activity journal can help you understand those subtle risk factors in your life that trigger an increase in your fatigue.

Staying within your limits gives you an advantage of being able to increase your output without penalty and follow your graded exercise program. And staying within your planned program and your limitations also will help to prevent the dreaded "wired but tired" feeling that comes from immobility, lack of refreshing sleep, and chronic fatigue. That wired but tired feeling often comes at the end of long days of severe fatigue where you have not adequately tired your muscles or your mind due to the fact that you simply cannot. You then are not physically tired enough to sleep, even though you have felt miserably exhausted all day.

So you have no excuses, the outline for staying within your limitations is summarized here:

- Don't start any activity if you feel fatigued. Only exercise when you feel rested.

- Always stop any activity before you have overdone it by doing only half of what you think you can do.

- Limit activities daily until you are sure you have an energy savings as evidenced by your increasing endurance.

- Don't force yourself to stick to plans. Instead, abandon them if you have any reservations.

- Prioritize and save unnecessary tasks for a later day.

- Ask for help from friends and family.

- Slow down, move slower, work slower, and rest in between activities.

- Wait until afternoon to exercise and consistently follow your graded exercise program.

- Extend your energy savings by switching activities before you get fatigued.

Mike is a 49-year-old computer programmer who became chronically ill after a flu-like illness. After four months of testing and uncertainty, his doctor finally gave him a diagnosis of CFS. By then Mike had cut down his hours at work to barely two hours a day and on some days was unable to come in at all. After receiving his diagnosis, he was disheartened to discover that there was no real medical cure for his debilitating condition and the most he could hope for were therapies designed only to improve symptoms. Mike decided not to accept that prognosis and proceeded to outline his plan for health restoration based on the healing principles of stress reduction, nutrition, rest, and exercise.

Mike discovered PEM early on, but he also believed the ancient Chinese proverb, "Worms will not eat living wood where the vital sap is flowing; rust will not hinder the opening of a gate when the hinges are used each day. Movement gives health and life. Stagnation brings disease and death." As part of a plan, he started to journal his activities and results including what made him feel worse or better.

As an avid hiker, Mike used walking as his primary exercise and soon realized that walking in the afternoon was more tolerable leading him to be able to increase his speed and distance over time. He did realize that extending his exertion on days he felt better only set him back that day or the next day. Mike realized that the expected reaction of becoming tired while exercising wasn't a gauge he could depend on, rather flares of fatigue and other symptoms were almost always delayed. For example, sometimes he felt great after a walk, but later on he felt punished by fatigue and pain that usually extended into the next day or beyond.

By adhering to pacing and graded exercise, Mike was able to build endurance and strength while avoiding deconditioning. Over the course of several years, he also realized that taking rest breaks while walking actually gave him a boost of reserve strength in both preventing PEM and the ability to increase intensity. Although Mike's total recovery from CFS took more than five years, he believes that using a systematic approach of pacing and graded exercise were an essential part of his healing process.

The Importance of Rest and Naps

There are no hard-and-fast rules in regard to napping and fatigue. Healthy people call the midday nap the "power nap." While the power nap is a great way to regenerate, it might not work for people who are very ill or very fatigued. For example, if you have a sleep disorder such as insomnia, you might find that daytime napping interferes even more with nighttime sleep. Because you may have problems with your circadian rhythm or other issues, such as achieving deep sleep, you should avoid taking daytime naps—particularly if they cause you to have trouble falling asleep at night or further disturb your nighttime sleep.

If napping doesn't interfere with nighttime sleep, you might actually need the additional rest; however, you should limit your nap to thirty minutes or less. And be careful not to nap late in the day because this can end up changing or interfering with your sleep wake cycle.

There is, however, one hard-and-fast rule about rest. You can reap the benefits of rest by simply stopping all activity, such as talking, reading, working, and even watching TV, and be still. Then, rather than actually sleeping, simply lying down in a horizontal position in a darkened and cool room for five to fifteen minutes several times a day might be sufficient to begin restoring your energy levels. You may have to experiment with which kind of rest is most restorative for you. However, just becoming horizontal at the onset of any symptoms can put those symptoms to bed.

The Least You Need to Know

♦ Having an informed and accepting attitude of your limitations during your recovery will help keep you on track without feeding any toxic negativity into the process.

♦ Pacing refers to the continual planning for rest, expending energy only within your limitations, and gradually increasing energy expenditure only when you have enough saved. Do only half of what you think you can do, continually evaluate your energy savings and level of endurance, and pull back as needed to get required rest.

♦ Too little activity or to much rest causes deconditioning, and that can be just another hurdle that you will have to overcome because it can drag you down further.

♦ Graded exercise is a planned exercise program that starts out slowly and increases in very small steps. This means that you stay within your plan even on good days when you feel like doing more. By staying within your plan, you are less likely to exceed your energy savings while you build strength and endurance.

♦ Plan to exercise in the afternoon rather than morning, begin with stretching exercises like yoga, and increase to include weight training; finally, when you have enough endurance include cardio and aerobics.

♦ Keep a written record to help you to see the amount of time and the types of activities you can do without experiencing post exertional malaise (PEM), which is the worsening of fatigue or other symptoms after exercise or activity. List activities that have minimal or no risk of causing PEM, those with moderate risk, and those that are absolutely "no can do" activities.

Sweet Dreams

In This Chapter

- ◆ Calculating your sleep requirements
- ◆ Do you have a sleep disorder?
- ◆ Dealing with insomnia
- ◆ Tips for shift workers
- ◆ How sleep deprivation hurts

Losing sleep means lost productivity and decreased mental abilities, pure and simple. But did you know that lost sleep also is associated with a higher risk of motor vehicle accidents; increased appetite leading to weight problems and obesity; increased risk of heart disease, diabetes, and hypertension; and increased risk of mood disorders and substance abuse? Whew! Overuse of drugs like stimulants, sedatives, and alcohol cause you to have highs and lows that interfere with the body's normal ability to regulate during wake and sleep.

Sleep disorders can be a chronic nightly problem that adversely affects your daily functioning and behavior, worsens any medical problems you may have, or causes new health problems. You can have sleep deprivation because of emotional disorders, physical disabilities, or even lifestyle. With time, effort, and commitment to making the necessary lifestyle changes, along with treatment, you can conquer those sleep demons and get the health-restoring sleep you need.

The consequences of burning the candle at both ends resulting in chronic sleep deprivation can be far worse than simply being tired and off your game. Getting your required sleep every night and paying off your sleep debt can keep you healthy, improve your quality of life, and help win your fight against fatigue.

Your Personal Sleep Requirements

How much sleep is enough? The reality is that there isn't one magic number that applies to everyone and the number of hours you require might be different from your friends, co-workers, or even those you live with. Your personal sleep requirements depend on a number of factors.

The first factor is your basal sleep need, or the amount of sleep your own body needs to get regularly to perform at its optimum. Most healthy adults' basal sleep requirement is seven to nine hours. Although some people believe that older adults need less sleep, the truth is that it's not a need for sleep but the ability to sleep that worsens with age. And researchers now believe that the reason older people have problems sleeping and feeling sleepy during the day is due to illness and poor sleep habits.

Second, you have to factor in your sleep debt, which is the cumulative amount of sleep you have lost over time due to your poor sleep habits, illness, nighttime awakenings, and other causes of lost sleep. Factoring in your sleep debt to figure out your present sleep requirement is where it gets tricky.

For example, you might be meeting your basal sleep need for a night or two or three in a row but still have not recouped your unresolved sleep debt. So, the fact that you feel sleepy or fatigued after a good night's sleep might be throwing you for a loop. Not waking up refreshed after a good night's sleep can be due to numerous causes, but taking care of your sleep debt might just put one cause to bed.

A small amount of sleep debt—that is, debt that has not caused you to have complete burnout—can be paid off eventually by returning to regular sleeping and waking times and getting your required amount of sleep. How long it takes to pay off your debt depends on how sleep deprived you are, so give it time after you begin to put in the hours.

In The Know
"There is strong evidence that sufficient shortening or disturbance of the sleep process compromises mood, performance, and alertness and can result in injury or death. In this light, the most common-sense 'do no injury' medical advice would be to avoid sleep deprivation." —*Sleep researchers Michael H. Bonnet and Donna L. Arand*

So, let's start by taking a look at your sleeping habits. Do your retiring and awakening times constantly vary by about two to four hours? Do you spend time in bed while not asleep (that is, tossing and turning)? Does the amount of sleep you get each night vary by more than one or two hours? Is the quality of your sleep poor and do you nap or require naps? Answering yes to most of these questions indicates that you have a problem with sleep habits (called sleep hygiene) or you may have a sleep disorder.

Look at how many hours of sleep it typically takes to make you feel productive, healthy, and happy. Do you have weight problems, medical conditions, or sleep problems; depend on caffeine for energy; or ever feel sleepy when driving? These can indicate that you might not be getting enough sleep, if you have healthy sleep habits, or if you need to see your doctor or a sleep specialist for some help.

Getting adequate sleep every night is as important as eating a healthy diet and needs to be made a priority in your life. It's one of the most basic requirements in winning your fight against fatigue.

Sleep Disorders

There are many types of sleep disorders as well as causes. Some may be easily treated, however, there are others that you need to make your doctor aware of.

Look over this list of symptoms. If you experience one or more of them, please discuss them with your doctor:

◆ Gasping for breath or periods of not breathing during sleep that is reported by others

◆ Memory problems/difficulty concentrating

◆ Depression or irritability

◆ Morning headaches

◆ Leg discomfort occurring at night

◆ Fatigue/excessive sleepiness

◆ Trouble falling asleep, waking frequently during the night, waking and not being able to fall back asleep, or waking unrefreshed

◆ Loud snoring

◆ Movement of your arms or legs during sleeping that is reported by others

◆ Weakness and/or loss of muscle strength sometimes in response to a strong emotion

◆ Sleepwalking/sleep talking

◆ High blood pressure

◆ Excessive daytime sleepiness, frequently falling asleep at inappropriate times (during meetings, while driving)

Sleep Apnea

People with sleep apnea stop breathing frequently—sometimes hundreds of times while sleeping and often for a minute or longer. See Chapter 2 for an explanation of the three types of sleep apnea: obstructive (the most common), central, and mixed.

Both main types of sleep apnea—central and obstructive—have symptoms of loud, frequent snoring, snorting, or choking; frequent episodes of not breathing (apnea); and excessive daytime sleepiness. Sleep apnea tends to affect overweight people, although it can affect people in all weight and age groups, and occurs more often in men than women. It is accompanied by hypertension, daytime sleepiness, decreased quality of life, and even a history of motor vehicle accidents due to mental impairment. Symptoms of sleep apnea are most often noticed by a family member who typically leads the person affected to seek medical help.

Your best bet to treat obstructive sleep apnea is to lose weight. Added adipose tissue deposits in the airway tend to cause or aggravate airway obstruction at night.

Because sleep apnea is seen more in overweight people, the most effective long-term treatment for obstructive sleep apnea is to lose weight. For those unable to lose weight, there are effective treatments.

In The Know

"If you treat people with high blood pressure and sleep apnea, or heart failure and sleep apnea, the measures of blood pressure or heart failure are significantly improved. There is good evidence to think there is a cause-and-effect relationship between hypertension and sleep apnea."

—Virend K. Somers, M.D., Professor of Internal Medicine in the Division of Cardiovascular Diseases at the Mayo Clinic in Rochester, Minnesota

---

A common treatment for sleep apnea is the use of a continuous positive airway pressure (CPAP; pronounced see-pap) machine. This machine delivers pressure to the airway with compressed air by a mask that covers the nose or the nose and mouth. The compressed air that flows into the airway supports the tongue and prevents airway obstruction. CPAP needs to be used at night and during naps.

Some people are prescribed a BIPAP (pronounced bi-pap) machine. BIPAP provides two levels of pressure: higher pressure when inhaling and lower pressure when exhaling. Because it's more like normal breathing, some people find it more comfortable.

Restless Legs Syndrome

The cause of Restless Legs Syndrome (RLS) is unknown, although it seems to run in families. RLS also might have some correlation with anemia or low iron levels; kidney failure; diabetes; Parkinson's disease; peripheral neuropathy; pregnancy (particularly during the last trimester); medications including antinausea drugs (prochlorperazine and metoclopramide), antiseizure drugs (phenytoin and droperidol), antipsychotic drugs (haloperidol and phenothiazine derivatives); cold and allergy medications; caffeine; alcohol; and tobacco use.

According to the International Restless Legs Syndrome Study Group, the four basic criteria for diagnosing RLS are:

- A desire to move the limbs, often associated with uncomfortable sensations
- Symptoms that worsen or are present only during rest and that are partially or temporarily relieved by movement or activity
- Restless movement of limbs
- Worsening of symptoms at night

The diagnosis of RLS is subjective and is made largely on the descriptions of the symptoms, medical history, family history, and medication use. Tell your doctor how often you experience symptoms; how long they last; their intensity; your sleeping habits; and about any sleep loss, fatigue, or sleepiness during the day and any disturbance in day-to-day functioning. Your doctor also might do some lab tests to rule out anemia, low iron stores, diabetes, and kidney dysfunction.

You might have tests to measure electrical activity in your muscles and nerves and to evaluate muscle activity in your legs to assess any possible damage or disease in the nerves and nerve roots (called peripheral neuropathy and radiculopathy). Or you may undergo sleep studies that record brain waves, heartbeat, and breathing to rule out periodic limb movement disorder (PLMD)—repetitive jerking or cramping of the legs during sleep. Your doctor might then diagnose RLS when all other causes of your symptoms are excluded.

Treatment of RLS is focused on relieving symptoms. For iron deficiencies, your doctor will most likely give you supplements in the form of iron, folate, and magnesium. Maintaining regular sleeping hours can reduce symptoms. If you find that your RLS symptoms decrease in the early morning, changing your sleep patterns might allow you more refreshing sleep. While regular moderate exercise improves sleep, excessive exercise often aggravates RLS symptoms. Hot baths, leg massage (this is where a portable massage unit comes in handy), heating pads, and ice packs sometimes alleviate the symptoms. Daily yoga exercise improves circulation to your lower extremities, often providing relief.

Some dietary and supplement suggestions that might help to alleviate RLS symptoms include: vitamin B complex supplements, including garlic in the diet, getting 400 I.U. per day of vitamin D, and eating foods that are rich sources of the nutrient folate (such as asparagus, spinach, and kale juice). Be sure to consult with your doctor before taking any supplements.

Energy Bar _____

RLS symptoms often improve with dietary modifications, particularly a diet that includes frequent, small, sugar-free, high-protein meals; frequent snacking; and a bedtime snack. This diet requires eliminating refined flour, caffeine, and alcohol and eating a diet of whole grains, nuts, seeds, fresh fruits and vegetables, and fish.

Medications to treat Parkinson's disease (dopaminergic agents) can reduce RLS symptoms and PLMD and usually are the first choice. However, even though they initially help to lessen symptoms at night, after a while the symptoms typically begin to develop earlier in the day. This effect can be less likely with dopamine agonists such as pergolide mesylate, pramipexole, and ropinirole hydrochloride. Ropinirole is the only medication approved by the FDA to treat moderate to severe RLS.

Benzodiazepines (clonazepam and diazepam) may help partially alleviate mild or intermittent symptoms for a more restful sleep. Opioids (codeine, propoxyphene, and oxycodone) might be prescribed for severe symptoms to promote relaxation and alleviate pain, but they also can cause nausea, vomiting, and dizziness and carry a risk of addiction.

Anticonvulsants (carbamazepine and gabapentin) can decrease creeping and crawling sensations but also can cause fatigue, dizziness, and daytime sleepiness.

Along with side effects, medications that are taken on a regular basis can become less effective over time (this is called augmentation) if this happens, talk to your doctor about different medications you can try.

Insomnia

Insomnia is difficulty falling asleep, staying asleep, or both and is a symptom that affects all age groups; women are affected more often than men, and occurs more often with age. The most common trigger of acute short-term insomnia is stress. Acute episodes of insomnia can have psychological causes (anxiety, stress, and depression) or physical causes (pain, congestive heart failure, chronic obstructive pulmonary disease, and degenerative diseases like Alzheimer's disease). If acute episodes of insomnia are not addressed, it can result in a chronic problem because you begin to worry about your ability to sleep and the problem then dominos.

People who travel frequently, shift workers, older persons, teens and young students, and pregnant and menopausal women all are in a high-risk group to experience insomnia.

Certain medications also have been linked to insomnia; these include prescription and over-the-counter (OTC) cold and asthma medications and high blood pressure medications. In addition, caffeine and nicotine are known stimulants that disrupt the ability to sleep. Alcohol is not only associated with sleep disruption, but is also a cause of nonrefreshed sleep (fatigue).

When insomnia lasts longer than four weeks or interferes with your ability to function, it's time to seek help. Your doctor will need to evaluate and treat any medical or psychological illnesses that are causing or contributing to your insomnia, including sleep disorders, pain, depression, anxiety, or other mental health problems or physical conditions. Behavioral techniques improve chronic insomnia in the majority of people without risks and side effects of medications. Self-help techniques to improve sleep include the following:

- Improved sleep habits and environment (sleep hygiene)

- Relaxation techniques and stress management

- Acupuncture and massage

- Cognitive-Behavioral Therapy

- Herbal remedies and nutritional supplements

Sleep hygiene is part of a well-rounded program to improve your ability to sleep. Like other fatigue interventions, sleep hygiene requires some effort and dedication on your part and the results you get will depend on the amount of effort you put into it. Use the same bedtime routine every night. Consistently go to sleep and get up at the same time, and make getting enough sleep a priority in your life. It's fairly obvious that you should get to bed at a time that will ensure you get your necessary amount of sleep. If you need eight hours of sleep and you have to get up at six in the morning then go to bed at ten or a few minutes before hand. However, some insomniacs mistakenly go to bed too early, and thus the time they spend tossing and turning becomes a negative conditioning related to sleep.

You want to associate your bed with rest and relaxation, not stress, work, or even mind-stimulating activities like watching TV. So, if you are in the habit of working or dealing with other stressful problem-solving work in bed, find another spot to do that and do it in the morning, not before you go to bed. Also, move the TV out of your bedroom and use your bed only for sleep and sex—don't even read in your bed. Turning off the TV and computer two to three hours prior to sleeping can help because both can stimulate your mind. Try to read something spiritual or soothing like poetry to help you to relax.

Take a hot bath ninety minutes before bedtime, but not after that time because your body needs the cooldown period to relax and fall asleep. A hot bath raises your body temperature, but it's a drop in body temperature that can leave you feeling sleepy.

Eat your last meal at least three hours before you sleep and avoid sugars for bedtime snacks. A meal raises your blood sugar too high, inhibits sleep, and later when your blood sugar drops too low you might wake up and not be able to fall back asleep. Instead, have a snack that contains the amino acid tryptophan (a natural relaxant), such as milk or turkey, along with a small piece of fruit or other complex carb to help the tryptophan cross the blood-brain barrier. Avoid eating foods that you might be sensitive to because the resulting indigestion or heartburn will keep you awake.

Vigorous exercise, caffeinated beverages, smoking, alcohol and sleep just don't mix. All of them are stimulating and should be avoided in the evening. Any fluids a couple of hours before you retire can cause your bladder to wake you in the middle of the night. Try setting a cutoff point after which you will not eat, drink, smoke, or exercise and vary it as needed depending on how much effect you find it has on your sleep.

Make your bedroom as dark as possible, and if you can't get it dark enough, wear an eye mask. Some people sleep better wearing socks to bed because feet have the poorest circulation and cold feet often keep you awake or wake you up. Other people are more comfortable without socks, but everyone should keep their bedrooms at a cool temperature, preferably around 68 degrees.

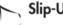 **Slip-Ups**

Don't have emotional conversations in the two hours before bed ... that can include talking on the phone. Something in your conversation might stimulate your mind to start thinking and that will only contribute to hyping you up and lead to those pesky racing thoughts.

Go ahead and indulge in that super-comfortable pillow and even high-end sheets if you can. And while you're at it, change your sheets as often as possible, ideally every three to four days. Clean sheets not only make you feel more pampered, but they also increase your comfort level by staying cooler and less itchy. This can be due in part to keeping the proliferation of dust mites down, which has an added benefit of reducing allergy symptoms (and fatigue).

Try using a white noise CD or a fan to create white noise in your bedroom at night because this can be soothing to your nervous system. There are also delta wave sleep-inducing CDs you can use. Delta is the brain wave associated with deep sleep. Buy a CD player that has an auto-replay feature so the CD will play continuously through the night.

Any light at all during the night will disrupt your circadian clock and your ability to sleep, so keep lighted clocks out of your bedroom, face them away from you, or put a cloth over them. You also can buy a clock that requires you to push the top button for it to illuminate. An added benefit is that you don't have that convenient continual reminder of what time it is during the night, and you might find after a few nights that you've trained your brain not to care or worry about the time.

Learning mental and physical relaxation techniques to perform before bed will help you fall asleep more effortlessly. You can start to wind down by reading a book, taking a bath, or working a noncompetitive puzzle ninety minutes before sleep.

Or you can try more structured relaxation or stress management techniques such as progressive muscle relaxation. To do this, first tense your muscles and then relax them starting at the top of your body and working down. By the time you reach your toes, you should be very relaxed.

Try slow, deep abdominal breathing while focusing on your breathing in order to unwind. First, take a deep breath and hold it to relax your diaphragm; then exhale slowly. You also can try visual imagery relaxation or self-guided imagery by closing your eyes and imagining an activity or a place you find peaceful and calming.

Using a journal to put your thoughts down on paper before you sleep will help you to resist dwelling on them. You can also use the written word to release any anger and to write a to-do list telling your brain that, yes, you remember what you have to do tomorrow so you don't need a continual reminder in racing thoughts.

If you can't sleep, get up, leave your bedroom, sit in a darkened room (don't turn on a light), and do deep breathing and meditation till you feel sleepy; then return to bed. Try meditating on something other than your problems. Think of one thing that makes your life pleasant and meditate on that. Try also to train your mind not to think when you find your mind racing. When your mind starts to wander, refocus to one word such as *relax, relax* or *calm, calm* while you are deep breathing.

Acupuncture has an extremely calming effect on your nervous system because it stimulates chemicals in the brain to help you sleep. Chances are you don't have the skills or the needles to perform acupuncture, but you can do acupressure on yourself using finger pressure on the same body points acupuncture employs. Using several fingers over the following areas, apply steady pressure for one to three minutes:

◆ Above the nose, between your eyebrows, on the small depression at the level of your brows.

◆ The middle of the inner side of the forearm two-and-a-half finger widths from the wrist crease.

- The inside of the wrist crease in the same line as the little finger.

- The depression between your first and second toes, on top of the foot.

- Beginning at the tips of your toes, the distance one-third back toward your heel on the sole of your foot.

- Any point on your ears—either apply pressure or massage.

If you are lucky enough to have a willing partner to give you a massage, it can help you relax and promote sleep. Or you can use a portable massage unit to ease your tense muscles.

Bright light therapy is artificial light that is used to treat sleep problems associated with jet lag or shift work to simulate the effects of sunlight on the body's circadian (day/night) rhythms. Your internal clock is "set" by your exposure to bright light or sunlight. Light therapy can be used to augment your other sleep hygiene measures. The most common tool in light therapy is a light box that contains several tubes that produce a bright light. From a distance of about 18 to 24 inches, you are to face in the direction of the box but not looking directly into the light. You can work or read while your body is using the light to regulate your internal clock. Light boxes are available in a variety of makes, models, and prices.

Other bright light therapies come in the form of a desk lamp that can be used in an office setting, a light visor designed to be worn on your head, and a dawn stimulator that gradually makes a dark room brighter over a set period of time.

Isolated sleep problems sometimes become chronic because periods of insomnia can be incredibly anxiety-provoking and lead to stress and worrying about not being able to sleep, a sort of self-fulfilled prophesy. Cognitive-Behavioral Therapy (CBT) can help change your thinking about sleep, correct behaviors, and any erroneous assumptions or beliefs. If you have corrected your sleep habits and sleep hygiene but are still suffering from insomnia, it might help you to talk with a therapist about CBT.

For people with chronic insomnia, your best bet might be a combination of good sleep hygiene and the use of sleep supplements. Although prescription sleeping pills work in the short term, they can add to the problem with a risk of chemical dependency, tolerance, and even addiction.

Energy Bar

Get some sunlight everyday to help regulate your circadian clock and make you feel sleepy at night. Sunlight stimulates a gland in your brain (pineal gland) to produce melatonin, a hormone that regulates your sleep cycle.

def•i•ni•tion

Melatonin is a hormone made by the pineal (pronounced pin-ee-all) gland in the brain each night to help us sleep. Melatonin production decreases with age.

According to the American Academy of Sleep Medicine, the most popular supplement for insomnia is *melatonin*, a naturally occurring hormone that regulates the sleep-wake systems in your brains. Taking one milligram of melatonin thirty minutes prior to bedtime often decreases the time it takes you to fall asleep and prolongs sleep duration. To avoid any tolerance, don't use melatonin every night—try using it every third night.

Taking tryptophan supplements can increase your own natural production of melatonin production. For serious insomnia, try taking a low dose of melatonin (0.5 to 1 milligram) along with 500 to 1,500 milligrams of tryptophan thirty minutes prior to bedtime. These nutritional supplements can be purchased OTC.

Calcium and magnesium are mildly sedating. Because you need to take your daily calcium/magnesium supplements in divided doses so that calcium can be absorbed and the excess is not excreted, take one half of your calcium/magnesium supplement at bedtime.

Gotu kola is an herb used for insomnia that has been called one of the "miracle elixirs of life" from a legend whereby an ancient Chinese herbalist who used it lived for more than two hundred years. Try making a tea by using one teaspoon of gotu kola in a cup of hot water and covering and steeping the leaf or flowers for five to ten minutes (or if you're using roots, steep them for ten to twenty minutes); drink two to four cups a day.

Lemon balm is a calming herb used to reduce stress and treat anxiety, promote sleep, improve appetite, and ease pain and indigestion. To make tea, use one-fourth to one teaspoonful of dried lemon balm herb steeped in hot water; drink up to four cups a day. You can also take two to three milliliters in a tincture (alcohol- and herb-based solution) three times a day or 300–500 milligrams of dried lemon balm capsules three times daily or as needed.

Valerian is an herb used to ease insomnia, treat stress-related anxiety and nervous restlessness, and to help people sleep. It can take a few weeks before you feel the effects if you take valerian as follows an hour before bed. To make tea, pour one cup of boiling water over one teaspoon of dried valerian root and steep for five to ten minutes before drinking. To take as a tincture, use one to one and one-half teaspoons. If you're taking it as capsules, take 250–500 milligrams.

You can take a combination of 180–360 milligrams of valerian and 80–100 milligrams of lemon balm to improve sleep without feeling sedated during the day. A small percentage of people find valerian root stimulating, and in that case, you should use it during the day to help you sleep at night. Start with the lowest dose of herb to see how it affects you and increase gradually as needed, not exceeding maximum dose.

Medications that your doctor might prescribe include eszopiclone (Lunesta), zaleplon (Sonata), and zolpidem (Ambien) or other drugs such as tranquilizers (benzodiazepines) and sedating antidepressants. A prescription drug that stimulates melatonin receptors is called Ramelteon (Rozerem), which is approved by the FDA for difficulty falling asleep.

OTC antihistamines that are sedating, such as diphenhydramine (Benadryl), also can be used in combination with an OTC pain reliever such as acetaminophen to cause drowsiness while relieving pain that might be keeping you from falling asleep or staying asleep. Start with a small dose (25 milligrams) of diphenhydramine and work up to 50 mg (generally recommend 25 to 50 not 100 as side effects increment at that dose ok). If you find that you are drowsy the next day, decrease your dose or discontinue using it.

Never take more than four grams or 4,000 milligrams of acetaminophen in a twenty-four-hour period. Many OTC and prescription medications contain acetaminophen so be sure that you check the label of all your medications so you don't exceed the recommended daily dose. Doses that are higher than recommended have been associated with severe liver problems, including liver failure and death.

Dealing With Shift Work

Shift workers, like everyone else, need to make sleep a priority and understand the importance of sleep. But sleeping during the daytime is often difficult because it's counter to your natural circadian rhythm (sleep/wake-day/night cycle), it's light outside and sometimes noisy and hot, and most people are awake at that time. Your first step should be to avoid the morning sun by wearing sunglasses on the way home and avoid stopping to run errands. Sleep in the most isolated room in your home and make sure it's dark, cool, and quiet. Invest in blackout curtains or an eye mask.

Try to develop a routine, including setting a time to sleep, and sleep at that time even on days off. Make sure that your phone is turned off and that your family knows not to bother you. Limit your caffeine or stop caffeine all together.

Another tactic to try is to move your sleeping hours forward so that you are sleeping later in the morning or early afternoon and so you wake right before your shift starts. You might find this schedule to be more in synch with your natural rhythm and easier to adjust to because your brain associates the afternoon and evening hours more strongly with sleep.

Shift Work Sleep Disorder (SWSD) is insomnia or excessive sleepiness that is associated with a work period occurring during the normal sleeping hours. In order to prevent excessive sleep deprivation, try not to work more than four twelve-hour shifts in a row or five eight-hour shifts in a row. Shoot for at least forty-eight hours off between a string of night shifts and resist the temptation to do excessive overtime, including extending your night shift hours by coming in early or staying late. Avoid rotating shifts because it's easier on your day/night rhythm to stay with the same shift for a longer period of time before switching to another shift. People are more apt to adjust their circadian rhythm to a permanent night shift. Bright light therapy can also help with SWSD by regulating your natural melatonin levels and resetting your body's internal clock, helping you to be able to fall asleep during the hours that you are able to sleep.

Burning the Candle

Research has shown that as little as seven nights of sleep debt or losing three or four hours a night has serious adverse effects, including affecting your ability to process carbohydrates, manage stress, and maintain your body's balance of hormones and lowering immune function. Burning the midnight oil is potentially as damaging to your health as a sedentary lifestyle, poor nutrition, and even smoking.

In The Know

"Our society seems to place a moral value on sleeping as little as possible." "In Europe, people are less impressed by short sleepers. Here we're almost embarrassed to say that we are going to bed early. Saying 'I'm tired and I'm going to sleep' is viewed as being lazy."

—Eve Van Cauter, M. D., internationally known investigator in circadian rhythms and endocrine systems in normal and pathological conditions

---

Most Americans get only seven hours of sleep or less without ever attempting to work off their sleep debt. Although individual sleep needs vary and some people do require less sleep than others, the majority are for the most part still pushing themselves considerably beyond what is healthy.

Staying up half the night to study or work is not making you smarter or more productive, but is in fact decreasing your brain's ability to utilize glucose and thus impairing your critical thinking, memory, and mental sharpness. To top it off, burning the midnight oil causes your blood levels of cortisol to rise, which accelerates the aging process. Are you frustrated with your weight loss efforts? Consider that sleep deprivation has been shown to cause insulin resistance, increasing the risk of obesity. Is your blood pressure too high? Try getting enough sleep! In other words, staying up to work, study, party, or socialize doesn't make you more productive—it only causes sleep deprivation and sleep debt, and that can make you old, fat, sick, and dumb.

The Least You Need to Know

- ◆ Individual sleep requirements vary from seven to nine hours depending on factors such as how much sleep debt you have.

- ◆ Fatigue might be due to a number of treatable sleep disorders.

- ◆ Insomnia can be managed by good sleep hygiene, relaxation and stress-reduction techniques, Cognitive-Behavioral Therapy, supplements, herbs, and medications.

- ◆ Shift work typically takes more effort and planning to get required sleep, but it can be managed with sleep habits and good sleep hygiene that is specific to sleeping during the day.

- ◆ Sleep deprivation is linked to a number of health problems including obesity, hypertension, cognitive impairment, and accelerated aging.

Chapter 13

Good Health Is a Lifestyle

In This Chapter

◆ Changing your lifestyle

◆ Eliminating toxins

◆ Dealing with allergies

◆ Managing menopause for both sexes

◆ Quitting harmful habits

◆ Prioritizing your plan for healing

Some people do heal from illnesses for which doctors have given them no hope. Dr. Kenneth Pelletier of the University of California, San Francisco Medical School studied these people and the characteristics they shared to understand the common denominators that led them all to overcome great odds and recover. Each one of them had experienced deep change within their psyche, mind, or personality from the use of meditation, prayer, or other spiritual practice. They had all restructured and revised their interpersonal relationships to a more healthy balance. They had also changed their diets to get optimal nutrition so that they fed and did not stress their bodies. They understood the meaning and importance of the spiritual aspects of life and the balance with the material aspects. And none of them felt that recovery would be given to them; rather they believed they needed to earn it and that it would be a prize for a long, hard struggle.

The chapters in this book are a blueprint for you to refer to in order to plan necessary lifestyle changes. You've learned the importance of removing toxins from your food, and now the next step is to remove them from your life. Unfortunately, most people, and even reality shows, promote the boot camp style of change when it comes to personal change. The truth is that real change happens first when you stop, breathe, think, plan, and sometimes pray about what you need to do to change yourself, your habits, and your life.

Lifestyle changes are critically important in the process of healing. In fact, according to a pioneer in the study and treatment of Chronic Fatigue Syndrome (CFS), Paul Cheney, M.D., this is "easily the most important and often the least emphasized" part of treating fatigue states, including those that are disabling like CFS.

Toxic Lifestyles

A toxic lifestyle typically is one with a busy schedule and high-stress levels. If you throw in a diet of nutritionally deficient processed and fast foods; smoking; prescription, over-the-counter (OTC), and street drug use; a sedentary lifestyle; alcohol consumption; coffee addiction; and the thousands of toxic chemicals in household and personal products on top of the environmental pollution of air and water, all of this can add up to a very toxic life.

Some small changes can result in major improvements. Try removing televisions from your bedrooms and eating meals at the table instead of in front of the TV. Something as easy as that can be instrumental in improving your diet (you'll eat less at the table) while opening up the channels of communication within your family. Then limit the amount of time you spend watching TV as well as the time you spend on nonwork-related computer use so that you can use your time for healthier behaviors that involve the company of others.

Stop dieting! Yo-yo and crash dieting never works and is simply not healthy, particularly because most diets require you to limit or avoid certain vital nutrients. The diet culture we live in has been propagated by a marketing frenzy. It spins its wheels in toxins, relies on stimulants and medications, is overstressed, and doesn't really encourage eating real food. Please never diet again, but instead eat a diet of real whole foods, eliminate processed foods and diet soda, drink plenty of water, and get your necessary rest and relaxation. Maintaining a healthy diet and lifestyle is your best bet for permanent weight loss and for overall health.

Walk as much as you possibly can. You can increase the amount of steps you take every day by purposefully parking as far as feasibly possible from your work or the entrance of a store. Take stairs instead of elevators, and get up from your desk and walk for a few minutes at regular intervals.

Try This at Home

Today we are becoming aware that the overwhelming amount of chemicals used in products for feel good, smell good, and other conveniences may have a downside. Studies are slowly being released in the mainstream media on such things as possible future reproductive problems in babies caused by chemicals used in baby products. Thus, the yin of progress and technology appears to have it's yang of disturbance and imbalance.

Like most changes, including such things as global warming, we have a lot of debate. If you can't see immediate and specific problems caused by products you use everyday, how then do you know it's the cause of health problems you may have? Much of this book is about connecting the dots and looking at extremes and toxins that have added up to causing your fatigue. It's up to you to weigh the evidence and make choices. This section is going to give you more information on how to effectively begin to reduce your exposure to harmful toxins.

Avoiding *toxins* in our very toxic world includes changing certain lifestyle habits. You first must become aware and next practice methods to reduce your exposure of toxins by avoiding, eliminating, and replacing many of the products you use. There are many currently known as "green" companies that make chemical-free products for personal and household use. Unlike products of old that claimed to be *nontoxic* because the chemicals in their product wouldn't actually kill you if consumed, these new products are truly made with effective but chemical-free ingredients.

def•i•ni•tion

Toxins are known poisons that harm the body and usually cause unwanted side effects. The word **nontoxic** on products only indicates that a substance may cause little to no adverse reactions if you eat it or inhale it. It does not guarantee that the product is harm free.

Whenever you need to use a product that emits volatile organic compounds (VOCs), including such things as home hair color, you need to use it outdoors or with good ventilation along with fans—in some cases, you might need to wear a face mask. When you have your clothes dry-cleaned, find a place to hang them to air out so that you can reduce your exposure to perchloroethylene, the toxic chemical used in dry-cleaning. For all other environmental toxins, if you can smell it, you know you are absorbing it into your body via your lungs. However, you can't always smell VOC emissions, and that's why it's important to always be aware and cautious.

Some of the worst toxic offenders are those that come out of spray cans or bombs such as with pesticides. Instead, use baits and traps to get rid of pests because they do not cause the entire area you are treating to become toxic. They are designed so the pest enters the container with the pesticide and then takes it back to the colony or nest. Alternatives to insecticides are diatomaceous earth (don't use the swimming pool variety), B.T. (a microbial insecticide), insecticidal soaps, beneficial nematodes (good bugs that clean up the pesky ones), and Neem oil (a natural insecticide). For pet flea control, use alternatives such as enzyme shampoos, using a 50:50 mixture of white vinegar and water sprayed on the pet, weekly washing of pet bedding, and frequent vacuuming.

Drinking filtered or bottled water reduces your consumption of potentially carcino-genic chemicals that may be present in certain water supplies; these can include ele-vated amounts of chlorine and other health-damaging elements found in water, such as aluminum, fluoride, gasoline additives, pesticides, and mercury. If you can, have your water tested for harmful components and install a home filtration system if you find problems in your water.

Mold and other fungal toxins are a common cause of allergies, fatigue, and reduced quality of life and are found in some buildings, peanuts, wheat, corn, and alcoholic beverages. To decrease your exposure to mold, take the following steps:

◆ Make sure your home is well-insulated to decrease the growth of molds and a buildup of toxins.

◆ Limit or eliminate house plants whose soil can grow mold.

◆ Don't use a fireplace or wood-burning stove because mold is found on the bark of wood and burning wood releases a large amount of particulate matter and pollutants into your home.

◆ Be careful to remove standing water regularly (such as in self-defrosting refrigerators).

♦ Use an exhaust fan or open the windows in your bathroom after showers and baths.

♦ Don't let clothes sit in the washer; rather dry them immediately.

♦ Don't install carpeting or padding on a concrete or basement floor, don't sleep in damp or poorly ventilated basements, and cover any dirt basement floors with plastic sheeting.

Cleaning Up

The easiest way to reduce toxic exposure is to reduce or eliminate the use of harmful substances in and on your body and in your home. Many Green companies make toxin-free personal care and household products that work well, are safe to humans and the environment, and are biodegradable. At the very least, use unscented products so you can cut down on some of your toxic exposure.

Completely eliminate unnecessary products such as air fresheners, stain repellants, dryer sheets, fabric softeners, or other synthetic fragrances because they all have a double whammy of first polluting the air and second polluting your body.

Energy Bar _____

Drive with your windows up and with your car's air recirculation mode turned on to help prevent strong outdoor toxins from entering your vehicle interior.

Elimination Diet

Food sensitivity, like an allergy, causes an immune response in your body that often leads to leaky gut syndrome and other health issues that add to your fatigue. Sometimes food sensitivities and reactions can be extremely subtle. They may be symptoms of other conditions and lab testing is not always accurate or conclusive. When you suspect a food allergy or sensitivity, the best approach is to start with a food elimination diet.

To do this, first remove all the common problem foods from your diet for two weeks. These are typically milk and milk products, egg, all grains (corn, wheat, rye, oats, barley, rice), sugar, citrus, legumes, beans, peas, peanuts, beef, chicken, pork, apple, white potato, food colorings and chemical additives, yeast, chocolate, cola, processed and packaged foods, coffee, tea, and alcoholic beverages. Read all food labels carefully.

Because you need to avoid so many foods, including bread, try the following meal suggestions:

◆ **Breakfast:** Sweet potato slices, yams, strawberries, melon, allowed nuts, fresh or canned pineapple, bananas sprinkled with chopped allowed nuts, melon, mineral water, baked or broiled fish, lamb, olive oil, shredded coconut, and sea salt.

◆ **Lunch:** Lamb, allowed vegetables, pears, banana with ground nuts or almond butter, kiwi fruit, grapes, fresh almonds, fish, sweet potato slices, salad with oil and vegetables, cabbage, broiled snapper, and almonds.

◆ **Dinner:** Sweet potato, yam, lamb, any allowed meat, avocado, allowed vegetables, fresh fruit with shredded coconut, almonds, baked or broiled fish, baked squash, roast duckling, Cornish game hen, sea salt, chopped allowed nuts, and baked or broiled fish.

◆ **Snacks:** Pineapple slices, celery sticks with almond or sesame butter, peaches, grapes, raw vegetables, allowed nuts, banana sprinkled with crushed nuts, and sardines (packed in olive oil).

On the elimination diet you might have a sort of withdrawal and feel worse for the first week or so, but you will feel a dramatic improvement as your body detoxes from the offending foods and your GI tract function improves. After two weeks, gradually introduce one eliminated food every few days to pinpoint which foods are causing you problems. Generally, if you keep these problem foods out of your diet for a few months and then reintroduce them slowly, using them only once every week or so, you will find that your sensitivity will have decreased.

 Slip-Ups

If you are eating a diet of real whole food, a cup of organic coffee, a homemade sweet, or piece of dark chocolate will increase your quality of life. But the daily extreme use of sugar, alcohol, chocolate, and coffee has dire health consequences and will only increase your fatigue.

Of course, even if you don't have food allergies or sensitivities, it's a good idea to purchase organic produce to eliminate toxins in your food. By buying organic, you'll avoid ingesting pesticides while getting the benefit of the most nutritious food.

Remember Natalie the nurse in Chapter 4 whose extreme behaviors and toxic lifestyle lead to her developing CFS? After many years of illness she began to work on eliminating fatigue stressors. Four years later although her condition had improved by 80 percent, she was still sick. Natalie recalled she had once tested positive for a wheat allergy, but hadn't taken it seriously because she didn't have the GI problems commonly associated with wheat and gluten allergies. Given that her whole-food diet and overall fatigue stressor reduction didn't seem to be enough, she gave a shot at eliminating wheat from her diet. The results were astounding. Within days Natalie felt better than she had in years. Her chronic allergy symptoms disappeared over the course of the next three weeks. Natalie's remaining symptoms including muscle pain, headaches, and weakness, symptoms of hypoglycemia (crashing and burning), and brain fog disappeared. Her energy continued to improve and she eventually reached the 100 percent recovery she had so diligently worked for.

Sinus Irrigation

Sinus irrigation is a do-it-yourself home procedure for nasal and sinus health that was handed down from ancient yogis and today is recommended by doctors. Daily irrigation can be phenomenally successful at clearing post-nasal drip and preventing sinus infections and allergic rhinitis by moisturizing your nasal passages, clearing pockets of infection, and rinsing away allergens. Like brushing your teeth to prevent cavities, the regular use of saline sinus irrigation works to keep the inside of your nose and your sinuses healthy.

Irrigating your nasal passages and sinuses can be used as a treatment for chronic sinusitis and has been found in studies to be just as effective as medications. In fact, sinus irrigation can sometimes improve the fatiguing symptoms of pain, headache, bad breath, cough, and runny nose while decreasing the need for medications in people with frequent sinusitis.

For people with allergies and chemical sensitivity, sinus irrigation helps to rinse out the offending allergens from the nose and sinuses and helps to decrease or even prevent allergic reactions if used immediately after exposure to airborne allergens. Sinus irrigation has even been touted to help prevent colds! In essence, the regular use of sinus irrigation promotes good nasal health and increases sinus-related quality of life.

To prevent nasal tissue swelling and damage to the tissues, you need to use a salt concentration similar to that of your body (isotonic) for irrigation. You can buy commercial products or a solution that is often used for intravenous infusion—Ringers-Lactate—or you can make your own solution and store it in the refrigerator for up to two weeks.

Sinus Irrigation Fluid:

½ teaspoon salt

½ teaspoon baking soda

1 teaspoon white corn syrup (optional)

1 pint warm (not hot) bottled or filtered water

Using a soft rubber-tipped bulb syringe, stand over a sink or in the shower with your head forward, mouth open, and chin out. Insert the tip of the bulb syringe filled with the solution into your nose, stop breathing, and squeeze the solution into your nose—being careful not to swallow. If you need to swallow, stop and bend your head forward to allow the solution to run out of your nose. Repeat this on the other side; then blow your nose very gently, closing off one side at a time and blowing with your mouth open.

If you are bothered with allergens in the air, try irrigating your sinuses twice daily at first and then every day to every third day or after activities that involve exposure to allergens.

People with chronic sinus problems will find that a retail pulsating system is more effective at increasing sinus health. Pulsating systems work to improve the action of the cilia inside the sinuses whose movement works to drain mucous, decrease edema, and improve sinus drainage. Be sure to talk to your doctor or medical care provider before you try sinus irrigation if you have long-standing sinus problems.

Managing Menopause

Loss of muscle mass and decreased energy and virility in men are the gradual changes associated with decreased testosterone levels sometimes referred to as *male menopause*. The changes are often precipitated by such lifestyle habits as not getting the required sleep throughout life. It's believed that sleep is a factor that is critically important for maintaining normal hormone levels and in restoring growth hormones in the body.

Exercise is also a vital factor in maintaining internal balance. Typically, men who allow themselves to free-fall into older age without actively maintaining their bodies with proper diet, exercise, and sleep realize the effects of aging including chronic fatigue in a more profound way than men who work to maintain their health. Although some men truly have a treatable medical condition such as hypothyroid or other hormonal disorders, other men can step up hormone production and maintain normal hormone levels by quitting smoking, reducing alcohol consumption, getting enough exercise, eating a proper diet of real whole food, and getting enough sleep.

In The Know

"The reality is, things like sleeping—which is critically important to restoring growth hormones and allowing you to maintain normal hormone levels—and things like exercise—especially if you can do it for an hour a day—are incredibly important in changing your life cycle so that you start to behave like you're 20 years younger."

—Dr. Mehmet Oz, cardiothoracic surgeon, author, and known as "American's doctor" from frequent TV appearances including The Oprah Winfrey Show

---

Women have more sudden, sometimes more uncomfortable, and in some cases life-altering changes that occur in midlife during the time known as menopause. Like men, women also can rebalance their hormones without using drugs. Or they can augment the use of bioidentical hormones by taking high-quality supplements; eating a healthy diet; and maintaining a lifestyle that supports the endocrine system including avoidance of toxins, stress reduction, and getting necessary rest.

Soy has been heavily promoted for its so-called health benefits, including the relief of menopausal symptoms. However, some doctors discourage its overuse in breast cancer patients. Not everyone is gung ho about the benefits of soy, and some people believe there may be health-damaging effects from this refined, processed, and heavily promoted and marketed product. Compounds in soy have been found to interfere with thyroid function (goitrogenic) and to cause or promote cancer. This is an issue with two sides, those for and those against, but some health experts such as Andrew Weil, M.D., discourage the use of soy supplements.

Soy is one of those products that you need to research on your own and make a decision as to whether it is right for you.

Weeding Out Harmful Habits

Everyone has heard the statistics for the health effects of smoking, drinking, using drugs, drinking too much coffee, staying up too late, or eating too much, but many people still continue to indulge in their bad habits. The truth is that there is no one-size-fits-all approach that will work for everyone for every type of problem. Each problem has to be approached in a creative multisystem problem-solving way.

Harmful habits are for the most part an addiction because they are typically uncontrollable, something you are used to doing regularly, and sometimes something you really like doing. Some habits create cravings that perpetuate the problem and cause a person to feel and act in distressing ways.

Three weeks is typical of the time it takes to overcome a habit or create a new one. But quitting some things takes more than putting in the time. It can take first believing that you can overcome it, then finding the confidence that comes from developing other coping strategies, and sometimes seeking professional intervention.

Some habits like smoking and drinking are best broken by going cold turkey; others like bad eating habits need a more balanced approach of slowly eliminating the bad and replacing them with the good. Habits like workaholism or perfectionism can take a lot of time and effort to overcome, but the first step to breaking any bad habit is developing insight and understanding how the habit is harming you and your life. Then you can formulate a plan using some of the techniques outlined in this book such as Emotional Freedom Techniques (see Chapter 15), stress reduction, prayer, and mediation to help you deal with overcoming harmful habits.

Tips for Quitting Smoking

Your first step in quitting smoking is to think long and hard about the pros and cons of smoking. It sometimes helps to write them down. Include the dangerous diseases it causes like lung cancer, heart disease, stroke, and of course nagging fatigue. Don't forget to add what it does to your appearance, your teeth and skin, and your smell and how it impacts your stress level.

It might help your motivation to know that by quitting smoking you will decrease your risk of developing a myriad of tobacco-related illnesses. After fifteen years, your risk factor for coronary heart disease becomes the same as someone who has never smoked. Plus, it takes only two years to decrease your risk of heart attack to the same level as those who have never smoked.

Believing that you can quit is truly half the battle, and that's why you need to boost your coping abilities and increase your support system as part of your strategic plan. When you tell other people, you not only will have the additional support, but you will also have others beside yourself to answer to when you slip up. So don't keep it a secret—use all the help you can find.

While you are winding up to quit, first decide on a particular quit date and then ration your cigarettes to a certain number until you reach your quitting day. Changing brands while you are tapering down also can help you to like cigarettes less.

It's no secret that nicotine is a powerful, addicting drug that causes both physical and psychological withdrawal. To help with cravings, be sure you drink lots of fluids, particularly plain water or unsweetened herbal tea.

Drinking coffee, soda, and alcohol and using street drugs like marijuana will only increase your urge to smoke! So you might pack an extra health punch and give up any of those potentially harmful habits you have while you are at it.

Try to keep your blood sugar on an even keel and stay away from sugar and fatty food. Instead, munch on raw veggies and eat small, frequent meals. Exercise regularly with something that you can stick to and that's doable, like a walk around the block whenever you feel an urge to smoke.

Energy Bar

Get plenty of sleep when you are quitting smoking or any other bad habit by going to bed earlier than you would normally. In a sense, your body is recovering, so take advantage of the extra sleep as a healing tactic.

Try deep breathing as outlined in Chapter 15. When urges hit, change what you are doing and do something that requires mental exertion. Changing your daily habits, like where you eat, where you drive, and what you do after work all can help distract your mind.

Find someone to quit with so you can support and inspire each other. Make an appointment to get your teeth cleaned so that you can start out with a fresh clean mouth. Finally, take advantage of the two most popular and well-known support systems:

◆ SmokEnders claim to be "the Oldest and Most Successful Smoking Cessation Seminar Program Ever Devised." You can get the self-study course by calling 1-800-828-HELP (4357).

◆ 1-800-NO BUTTS is a free, confidential resource that says it will double your chances of successfully quitting smoking.

Cutting Down on Stimulants

Do you indulge in the occasional sweet or cup of coffee that you really enjoy and slowly savor? Or are you someone who buys the package of mini candy bars because you simply have to have your fix on a daily basis? Are you relying on coffee or sodas to wake up in the morning, to tide you over till lunch, and to get you through the evening? What about alcohol? Do you have to have your after-work drink in order to "relax?"

These sort of "have to have" relationships with caffeine, sugar, and alcohol are really addictions to stimulants, just like nicotine. It indicates a sort of self-inflicted chemical imbalance caused by the use of the substances themselves. Without the use of your substance, you feel fatigued and frazzled, headachy and apathetic, anxious and stressed. Ironically, using these stimulants only makes you feel worse due to the revolving door of addiction.

Using stimulants is not only energy depleting, but also causes anxiety; insomnia; and other uncomfortable symptoms like heartburn, irregular heartbeats, and headaches. If you believe you have an addiction or addictions, it might be time to put an end to them. You can quit stimulants and recover relatively quickly after only thirty days of not using. You'll have more energy and improved coping abilities.

Your first step in understanding your dependence is to record you daily intake for a few days. Take the time to keep a journal of how much and how often you consume coffee, tea, chocolate, sugar or other sweets, diet and regular soda, cigarettes, or alcohol. Make a note with each entry of why you are "using" and how badly you need to use.

You should not be drinking in excess of three cups of coffee or tea per day. For any amount over that, gradually reduce your consumption by cutting down by one cup per day every few days until you are down to three cups per day. A gradual taper is necessary to prevent symptoms of caffeine withdrawal: irritability, headache, tremor, inability to concentrate, nervousness, restlessness, and fatigue.

A word of wisdom: if it's hard to keep track of how many cups of coffee or caffeinated beverages you drink per day, you are drinking too much.

If you are looking for an alternative drink to replace your daily coffee, try green tea. Although it does have caffeine, the health benefits far outweigh the negative aspects of the caffeine it contains. Try switching over to green tea so you can make health gains while you are losing your coffee addiction; just be sure you don't start using the caffeine in green tea as a crutch throughout the day.

When you are off caffeine, or have at least cut down, choose another stimulant that you use regularly and cut down in a similar fashion. If you use sugar, then tapering off will give you added health benefits including weight loss that also will increase your energy. Try replacing one sugary sweet with something nutritious every day until you are off sugar.

The quickest way to cut down on sugar is to stop adding it to foods like coffee, tea, and cereal. Sugar is sugar, so if you are using raw sugar, turbinado sugar, or honey in excess, it's still just sugar to your body. Work on eliminating or reducing processed carbs such as bread, bagels, refined white flour pastas, and snacks that are all simple carbs and in essence just sugar. Do not get hooked into the hype of sugar-free or fat-free snacks because processed food all contains additives and calories. Beware of artificial sweeteners and other additives because they only increase your cravings for sugar and carbohydrates.

Limit fruit to two servings a day but completely eliminate drinking fruit juice. While fruit has fiber and other healthy intrinsic compounds, fruit juice is only pure sugar with only half the nutrients found in a piece of fruit.

Alcohol is in a significantly different league than caffeine and sugar because it can be deadlier in a different fashion. Because alcohol abuse can also have legal implications, you might need to get help if you feel you have a problem. In general, women should not drink more than one drink a day and men no more than two drinks a day. A drink is a 12-ounce bottle of beer, a 5-ounce glass of wine, or a 1.5-ounce shot of liquor.

Like nicotine, begin by writing your pros and cons for drinking and set a goal date to begin tapering or to quit entirely. Keep a record of your drinking for a few weeks to have some concrete evidence of what you are consuming, why you are drinking, and how you feel before you have the drink and how you feel afterward. When you reach your taper day, use the following tips:

◆ Don't keep alcohol at home.

◆ Drink slowly and take a one-hour break in between drinks.

◆ Never drink on an empty stomach and drink some water after a drink. Try to plan your drink with your meal.

◆ Don't drink just because other people are drinking, and if you feel pressure from others to drink, stay away from those people. People who are giving you a hard time about something like not drinking are not your friends.

◆ Stay active and make plans to do something that doesn't involve alcohol.

◆ Get support if you need to, ask your doctor for help, or talk to someone at your church. Many churches have recovery programs that are also good places to make alcohol-free friends.

Don't forget that it takes most people a few tries to quit any bad habit. And something as big as quitting drinking can take time, effort, and even getting professional help.

Setting Priorities

Setting limits, accepting limitations, and reordering your life to include healthy balance requires not just looking at necessary changes, but also understanding where each change or new behavior ranks in importance. The job of rebalancing your life needs to take precedence over all else—in fact, getting well is your job.

Take the passion that you've put into activities that might not have been healthy, such as overworking, overexercising, or being a perfectionist, and redirect that passion into your program for health. Put your requirements for optimal nutrition, rest, and exercise; stress reduction; relaxation; and having regular fun first.

Sleep and rest need to be your number one priority because that is the one activity that will give you the energy you need to address all the other aspects of healing. This will absolutely require that you stick to a regular bedtime regime, meaning you have to say no to some activities and to some people. It's also going to mean saying yes to leisure and to working stress reduction into your daily life.

Nutrition and supplementation are next on the list. Eating real, whole, preferably organic food and decreasing and eliminating toxins, stimulants, and sugar all need to be vital elements in your plan.

Remember balance, balance, balance! The rest of your plan requires changes in other areas depending on your issues and the changes you need to make. When you adequately feed and rest your body, you will have the inner resources you need to make other gradual changes toward health. Don't forget to be kind to yourself. If you are putting in the effort that is the best you can do.

The Least You Need to Know

◆ Healing requires cleaning up all aspects of a toxic lifestyle: a busy schedule and high-stress levels; a diet of nutritionally deficient processed and fast foods; smoking; prescription, OTC medication, and street drug use; a sedentary lifestyle; alcohol consumption; coffee addiction; toxic chemicals in household and personal products; and environmental pollution of air and water.

◆ Avoiding toxins in our very toxic world requires changing certain lifestyle habits by becoming aware and practicing methods to reduce your exposure of toxins by avoiding, eliminating, and replacing products made with chemicals.

◆ The best approach to dealing with food sensitivity is to first go on an elimination diet excluding milk, grains, eggs, most meats, citrus, processed food, sugar, alcohol, chocolate, and coffee from your diet for two weeks and then gradually introduce one eliminated food every few days to pinpoint which foods are causing you problems.

◆ Quitting smoking and drinking take a systematic approach of making a plan, getting support from friends and professionals if needed, and practicing healthy lifestyle behaviors.

◆ Stimulants like coffee, tea, chocolate, sugar or other sweets, diet and regular soda, cigarettes, and alcohol are all energy depleting. By tapering or stopping the use of one stimulant at a time, you can begin to increase your energy while decreasing your dependence on these false energy and energy-draining substances.

Chapter 14

Glass Half Full

In This Chapter

- A close-up on stress
- How stress pounds your body and mind
- Balancing your mind and body
- Tips to combat stress
- How prayer and meditation fit in
- Let the sunshine in

Stress has a well-deserved bad rap. People throw stress around and use it as an excuse for just about anything. The truth, though, is that most people still underestimate the damaging effects of stress.

Your health is like a savings account. Everything you do to benefit your health and to protect against the invaders of pathogenic organisms, stress, toxins, and deprivation is akin to making a deposit into your savings account. Everything you do to the detriment of your health is like making withdrawals from your account. If you continue making withdrawals without making deposits, you will be left with nothing in your account. The cumulative effect of day-to-day stress and fatigue stressors can add up to severe health consequences.

To maintain mind-body equilibrium and health, you need to balance work and play and get your necessary rest, nourishment, and exercise. Sound like a tall order? Healthy self-care is doable if taken in small steps, changing one habit and eliminating one stressor at a time before moving on to tackle another.

Using self-care techniques such as stress reduction, a method of healing called emotional freedom technique (EFT), prayer, and meditation all can assist you in keeping your health portfolio in the black. Getting daily sunlight also can give you a sunny disposition, help you sleep, and keep you healthy.

What Counts as Stress?

Dr. Hans Selye spent his life studying stress, and he defined stress as "the non-specific response of the body to any demand," and a stressor as "that which produces stress."

Stress provokes your body's systems to defend and protect against a perceived attack by reacting with a would-be, should-be protective response. Of course, you're usually not being attacked by lions, but injury, illness, and emotional and mental stressors all cause the same stress response. And so do positives in your life (also known as eustress) such as graduation, moving, getting married, having a baby, and career advancement.

In regard to fatigue, you need to dig deeper in the concept of stressors to include behaviors, habits, and lifestyles that create a burden on your body and mind. For the purposes of really understanding the damaging effects of these burdens, I call them *fatigue stressors*. We all have to deal with small amounts of mental and physical stressors that tax our mind-and-body systems. But over time, the cumulative effect of continual and excessive fatigue stressors becomes a toxic load that can result in chronic mental and physical fatigue.

def•i•ni•tion

> **Fatigue stressors** are a poor diet; dysfunctional relationships; inadequate sleep, rest, or nutrients; excessive behaviors; medical conditions including addictions, overuse of medications, and toxic lifestyle habits and choices; and environmental toxins. Too many fatigue stressors will eventually result in chronic fatigue.

Looking at the number fatigue stressors you have in the following list will give you a better idea of the host of factors that are stressing your immune system, central nervous system, and adrenal glands:

- ◆ Physiological stressors including low blood sugar, infections, diseases, illness, surgery, allergies, chemical sensitivity, obesity, and menopause.

- ◆ Emotional factors such as depression, anxiety, anger and rage, and trauma from the past.

- ◆ Environmental stressors including toxins; pollution; mercury; and brain poisons such as MSG, food additives, and chemical artificial sugars like aspartame and sucralose.

- ◆ Lifestyle risks such as a diet of junk, processed, or restaurant food; addictions; workaholism; a lack of conditioning; overexercise; over or undereating; perfectionism; chronic dehydration; coffee consumption; and using stimulants.

- ◆ Shift work, frequent travel, insomnia, sleep disorders, sleep debt, or sleep deprivation.

- ◆ Current and past medical treatments, including chemotherapy, radiation, and the overuse of prescription and OTC medication.

- ◆ Lack of support, feeling unappreciated, being abused or neglected, feeling countersupported, burnout, and toxic relationships.

Making you stress out about how much stress you have is not the intent of this list. Instead, helping you recognize your risk factors is the first step in dealing with the stressors. Then, making gradual changes is your best path to developing lasting healthy lifestyle habits.

Why Stress Kills

The reason stress is so damaging is because your body's response to stressors is a fight-or-flight reaction, or the physical, internal response to any perceived danger. Even though you are typically not in physical danger if your boss is screaming at you, his red face and bulging neck veins still alert your brain to activate your internal alarm system. So all stress, either psychological or physiological pressure, results in the release of stress hormones—primarily adrenaline and cortisol—in your body.

Stressors produce stress which, in turn, causes a cascade of physical events in your body. Adrenaline is activated to increase your heart rate and elevate blood pressure and energy supplies in your body. Cortisol is produced to replenish the sugar (glucose) level in your bloodstream, to boost the use of glucose by your brain, to lower your pain sensitivity, and to heighten your immune response.

Continual stress puts your body in a state of constant activation of the stress response system. This chronic stress response leads to sustained elevated levels of sugar in the blood, or hyperglycemia (another link in the chain that can cause you to develop type 2 diabetes); hypertension; and other harmful metabolic conditions such as increased cholesterol and hardening of the arteries (arteriosclerosis).

The continual stress reaction also eventually impairs the excitability of your nerve cells leading to atrophy of nerve cells in an area of the brain that is vital for spatial and verbal memory. This slows down your thinking and makes you even more vulnerable to everyday pressures, mental health problems, anxiety, and depression.

Chronic stress weakens the immune system so you can't fend off illness and infectious agents as easily and you will tend to get sick more often and stay sick longer. Stress weakens your muscle tissue, decreases your bone density, and leads to that telltale cortisol-induced bulge in your midsection.

In other words, chronic stress can be a killer. It's pretty well accepted that chronic stress contributes to or causes such conditions as stroke, cancer, depression, obesity, substance abuse, ulcers, irritable bowel syndrome (IBS), memory loss, autoimmune diseases (such as lupus), insomnia, thyroid problems, infertility, eating disorders, and chronic fatigue.

Bottom line, excessive and ongoing mental stress and fatigue stressors first distress your mind-body systems and distress not dealt with leads to disability (illness, fatigue). Then disability leads to damage that is not reversible. And because the ill effects of fatigue stressors accumulate over time, even doctors often fail to connect the dots to get to the bottom of your fatigue. Western medicine tends to compartmentalize and focus on just one organ or system, often missing the bigger picture. But we can't expect doctors to chip away at all the ways we are pounding our mind and bodies. Self-care is *our* job.

Maintaining Balance

A mind-body imbalance occurs when any part of your life is overextended, when you exceed the limits of human endurance, and when you lack rest periods between major stressors. The imbalance becomes even more extreme and less healthy over time when you add in any of the other stressors. You also lack fun and pleasure in your life. People aren't like the Energizer bunny—we can't just keep going and going and going.

Maintaining the internal equilibrium of your body for proper functioning involves each system staying within tolerable limits, known as homeostasis. Each bodily system reacts with internal modifications and depends on other systems to maintain its internal balances. Instability in one system affects the other systems.

Consider a rubber band that is continually overstretched. It reaches a point where it's no longer elastic, and it can then break. Your mind and body systems are the same in that they can be stretched only so far before they break. So, to be resilient and healthy, you need at the very least a continual supply of nutrients, exercise, and rest. The reason people often fail to grasp this is that they might have lived a life of excess and deprivation in overwork or overexercise, or they might have sleep debt and a poor diet, and because it has worked for them before. Thus, they fail to connect the dots when they become fatigued or ill. The truth is that, like the rubber band, they were able to stretch and bounce back in their early years, but later they lose that resiliency, that ability to adapt or bounce back.

The good news is that by working on eliminating fatigue stressors, you can in time reduce the distress and eliminate your fatigue. Even if you are diagnosed with a medical problem, you can live a healthier life with that diagnosis by eliminating toxic fatigue stressors. This means that, no matter what your state of health, if you gain control of all the fatigue stressors in your life, you can reverse, slow down, and prevent other problems—including fatigue.

Slip-Ups

Don't neglect your inner voice when it tries to tell you your body is sick and tired or stressed. Knowing and staying within your boundaries and personal limits can help you relieve the stress of unrealistic or unattainable goals.

Stress-Reduction Techniques

There are many ways to deal with stress, some healthy, some not. Instead of using unhealthy behaviors to self-medicate, such as alcohol and drug abuse, smoking, or overeating, you can use stress-reduction techniques for a temporary reduction in your stress level.

Stress-reduction techniques are used to control and counter the immediate physical effects of stress on your body. The techniques you chose to practice should vary with the type of stress you are experiencing. Your results will depend on your dedication to reducing stress and how much you practice. It doesn't matter whether you are at your desk or sitting at home; you can practice the following techniques anywhere.

Relaxing Your Mind and Body

Progressive muscular relaxation is a stress-reduction technique whereby you simply tense muscles as tightly as you are able, hold them tensed for several seconds, and then relax the muscles as much as possible. Starting with the muscle groups at the top of your body (such as upper arms and shoulder by squeezing shoulder blades together, hands by making a fist, forearms by pressing your palms together firmly) and working down will help you to relax your entire body.

Energy Bar _____

Try using progressive muscular relaxation and deep breathing to relax and prevent some of the damage from stress when adrenaline is pumping.

Deep breathing consists of a series of deep, slow breaths. First, breathe in slowly through the nose, hold the breath, and then exhale through the mouth.

A third method of stress relief is visualization. Close your eyes, relax your muscles, do some deep breathing, and picture a serene or ideal location in your mind. Take a moment and try it now. Don't you feel better?

Visualization also can use mental pictures of packing up worries and locking them away or throwing them off a bridge, or simply picturing stress flowing out of your body. Mental stress-reduction techniques such as visualization are useful when emotions are driving your stress.

One healing aspect inherent in these techniques is that the level of concentration they require takes your mind away from the stressor for at least a few minutes.

Each day, take some time to practice the following breathing, stretching, and visualization exercise:

1. Lie on your back on the floor; loosen any tight clothing.

2. Relax as much as possible and exhale fully; then inhale slowly through your abdomen, up to your ribs, and then your chest. Hold the breath briefly.

3. Exhale fully and repeat. Breathe normally for a few breaths; then repeat the deep-breathing exercise.

4. While breathing normally, raise your arms above your head and stretch them away and up. Return your arms to your sides.

5. Take a deep breath and stretch your legs and feet downward and relax.

6. Take a few seconds to feel the effects of your deep breathing and stretching on your body; then sit up very slowly.

7. Stand up and slowly bend backward as far as is comfortable without straining; then bend forward, followed by a side-to-side bend.

8. Sit down in a chair and close your eyes. While breathing normally, take a few minutes to notice sounds including outside noises and the sound of your breathing and how your body feels after stretching.

9. Continue quietly breathing for five to ten minutes, using the time to visualize stress flowing out of your body and healing light filling your body with each breath.

It takes fifteen or twenty minutes to learn and practice these techniques at first. After some practice, you might find you need only a few minutes to achieve the benefits of stress reduction, such as slowed breathing and heart rate, reduced anxiety, and a sense of relaxation and calm.

Ridding Yourself of the Negative

Nip those negative thoughts! Thought awareness is a proactive technique you can use to counter your negative thinking by purposefully thinking of a certain stress, identifying your negative thoughts, writing them down, and then letting them go. By taking the time and effort to identify those toxic thoughts, you can thereby work on putting an end to them by challenging their reality. Are you really the loser that your thoughts are saying you are, and would you expect similar condemnations from your friends? Are your thoughts rational and realistic? Or are you simply creating disaster scenarios in your mind?

Events that you place a significant importance on can increase your stress level, particularly when they include money, groups of people, competition, and being evaluated or judged. In cases where you feel your merit or finances are on the line, assuring yourself that your best is all you can do can decrease the mental pressure of important events.

If you have not solidified plans, done the work you need to do, or problem-solved to handle any potential plan B, then you should refocus your energies to do the necessary work rather than beating yourself up. Remember that you cannot control other people or what they say, and if they react unfairly to you, it's best to just think of it as their problem and not yours.

You also can replace negative thoughts with rational thoughts and affirmations or positive thinking. Affirmations are a time-tested method for improved self-confidence and changing destructive thinking habits. Instead of telling yourself you can't, tell yourself how much you have prepared, how hard you have worked, how skilled you are, and how ready you are to face any challenge. Of course, these sorts of affirmations have to be realistic, and you have to have done the work and be prepared in order to be confident in your real abilities.

By being prepared and focusing on your ability and your skillful performance, you can decrease the magnitude of the importance of the event in your mind. Uncertainty or lack of information often produces anxiety. Ask for clear instructions, get necessary itineraries, and ask for clarification and additional information to help set your mind at ease.

Taking It Easy

Incorporating stress reduction into your daily life can help prevent that continual feeling of white-knuckling through life and can help you ease up on the daily grind. Enroll in a yoga or Tai Chi class. Try to add beauty to your life with a nice table setting when you eat, flowers in your home, or treating yourself to other things you enjoy. Plan for enjoyable activities in your life, even planning a few minutes here and there just to rest and relax.

Slow down! Try doing everything a little more slowly and more deliberately. Instead of eating at your desk, take the meal breaks you deserve and enjoy your food. If at all possible, go outside during the day, if even for just a short walk or to sit in the sun.

Practice stress-reduction techniques whenever you begin to feel those telltale signs of stress, such as muscle tension, a racing heart, and sweating. Take frequent breaks from your work to relax and stretch your muscles. Remember to be as nice and gentle to yourself as you would want a friend or spouse to be. Take note of times at which you might be beating yourself up so that you can make the effort to stop those self-defeating behaviors.

Getting to the root of any problem is always the longest-lasting and most effective remedy for stress relief, and that includes nipping those things in the bud that are causing you continual stress. Start by working on healing your body and staying healthy with a regular exercise program, a healthy diet, regular sleep, reducing or eliminating alcohol intake, and stopping smoking.

Emotional Freedom Technique

That old expression "you'll feel better in the morning" really just doesn't apply when you wake up fatigued day after day. Waking up over and over not feeling rested can, in time, lead to feelings of defeat, frustration, and fear and can easily snowball into more negative thinking and lead to even more emotional and physical problems. Sometimes it's hard to figure out what came first, your depression or your negative pessimistic thinking. You know how damaging negative thinking can be, but stopping it is sometimes a challenge.

Negative emotions and thoughts are bad habits that can result in or worsen all mental problems. Negative thinking and its effects (including mental and emotional problems), and distress can be controlled, managed, and undone with the practice of emotional freedom technique (EFT). EFT is in essence a psychological acupressure technique that combines clinical psychology with elements of Eastern medicine and applied kinesiology to change and balance the strong relationship between your body-energy system and your thoughts and feelings.

The basic concept of EFT is that it removes blockages and constrictions in the energy flow, resulting in the elimination of stress, fear, and many other negative emotions that are thought to damage the body and weaken the immune system.

EFT uses the same energy meridians as traditional acupuncture that has been used to treat physical and emotional ailments for more than five thousand years. You don't need needles with EFT or extensive schooling; rather you use an easy technique of tapping with the fingertips on specific meridians while thinking about your negative thought or emotion and voicing positive statements. By practicing EFT, you will progress toward clearing that specific emotional blockage from your body's energy system.

To perform EFT, you need to learn the locations of the meridians or tapping locations, how to tap, and how to formulate your positive affirmations. The basic EFT recipe can be learned in just a few minutes, and after following the written sequence a few times, memorizing it is quick and easy. After a couple of tries, you can generally do the entire sequence in one or two minutes. EFT is centered on a single phrase: "even though I have this (insert negative thought or emotion), I deeply and completely accept myself," while tapping or rubbing certain defined meridian points on your body.

You can find an EFT practitioner online or can download the free basic manual at www.emofree.com and learn it yourself. EFT is gaining popularity with both alternative and integrative medicine practitioners for the treatment of anxiety disorders, phobias, weight loss, insomnia, and other health- and performance-related issues. EFT is so easy to do after it's learned that you can use it as a tool for healing just about any condition, mental/emotional problem, or mind-body imbalance.

In The Know

"I have found EFT to be an exceptionally effective and rapid-acting method to help patients overcome fears, cravings, and negative emotions. I often use it early in the process of therapy to treat the whole person. EFT definitely enhances the course of recovery by dealing with underlying emotional issues while I am focusing on physical and biochemical concerns."

—Roger Billica, M.D., FAAFP. *Former NASA Chief of Medical Operations. Internationally recognized in the field of preventive, integrative, and space medicine.*

Because EFT does not require rehashing painful events and emotional traumas to heal negative emotional states, it's an effective yet gentle method of restructuring healthy thinking and doing away with emotional distress.

Prayer and Meditation

Prayer and meditation are forms of self-care that are proving to have beneficial effects on the treatment of many conditions including drug addiction, depression, chronic pain, anxiety, insomnia, and PMS. These beneficial effects have been demonstrated in studies including those by Dr. Herbert Benson, president of the Mind-Body Medical Institute of Boston's Deaconness Hospital and Harvard Medical School. According to Dr. Benson, "Health is like a three-legged stool, and is supported by three types of treatments: pharmaceuticals, surgery, and self-care. Most of us believe that we need only two of these legs, and neglect our own self-care."

While prayer might have a placebo effect, the results of clinical studies show that those who pray have an improved ability to cope with any illness, are less likely to become ill, and more likely to recover from illness and surgery.

Prayer and meditation can improve immune function because of their effect on stress reduction. The inner peace that results from both practices has additional effects of reducing levels of stress hormones, decreasing feelings of anxiety, and in turn boosting immune function.

Praying for the healing of others (distance healing) is considered a form of alternative medicine because it's thought that caring, empathic, and compassionate feelings can actually encourage healing.

More than one hundred medical schools in the United States offer classes in faith and medicine because studies have shown that doctors praying with their patients and encouraging prayer can improve the outcomes of medical and surgical interventions. And prayer is taking place in mosques and ashrams, in healing rooms and prayer groups, in e-mails, in homes and schools, and at work by countless people all over the world. Schools like Stanford University teach meditative relaxation in their Arthritis Self-Help course as part of a comprehensive self-care program to control pain and learn to cope more successfully.

There's something about connecting to a higher power and calming the mind that has been used since the beginning of time. It could be believing there's something or someone bigger than yourself or the discipline of taking the time and effort—or there might be no rational explanation for the benefits of prayer and meditation. But both are here to stay.

Meditation and prayer are popular compliments to Western and alternative medicine that work to decrease negative thoughts and increase positive mindsets to assist in healing and improve quality of life by instilling a positive sense of well-being. Both require being still in some manner and being quiet. Either one can be done without any formal instruction, but both have volumes of information written about different methods and types that you can research and study. The best way to begin is to just stop what you are doing and sit in quiet reflection. You can then discover different ways to develop skills and to progress.

Sunlight Requirements

With all the skin cancer concerns, you might be hesitant to spend a lot of time in the sun. However, it might just be what you need to feel better. Vitamin D is produced by your body when natural sunlight contacts your skin. You need vitamin D for optimal health and to prevent conditions such as osteoporosis, depression, prostate cancer, and breast cancer. Because vitamin D deficiency impairs insulin production, it's also a factor in diabetes. Obesity impairs the utilization of vitamin D, so if you are obese, you need more sunlight exposure and more supplementation with vitamin D.

Fibromyalgia and vitamin D deficiency both have similar symptoms of aches, pain, and muscle weakness. It could be, then, that those with fibromyalgia are in fact suffering from a vitamin D deficiency.

Energy Bar _____

If you use sunscreen, try getting ten to fifteen minutes of sunlight a day without sunscreen to get your day's worth of vitamin D.

Natural sunlight can't penetrate glass, so your skin can't generate vitamin D when you are sitting in your car or at home in front of a window. And it's next to impossible to get the vitamin D you need in your diet, so you have to get it from the sun and, if needed, with additional supplementation. If you have dark skin pigmentation, you need approximately 20 to 30 times more sun exposure than a light-skinned person to produce the vitamin D you need.

It's thought that sunburn, together with excess omega-6 fats in your diet, increases your risk of skin cancer. In other words, your plan to lay out and bake in the sun while eating a burger and fries for lunch might not be such a good idea. But eating those superantioxidant foods such as tomato paste, pomegranates, and blueberries does increase your body's ability to deal with sunlight without burning. We're talking a reasonable amount of sun exposure here. And if you have chronic vitamin D deficiency, you can't reverse it overnight; rather you need months of regular sunlight exposure along with vitamin D supplements to rebuild your bones and nervous system.

The best approach to get your necessary vitamin D and other sunlight health benefits is to get your necessary dose of sunlight every day but to limit your sun exposure so that you avoid getting sunburned. Try getting some early morning sunlight when the temperature is cooler for the beneficial effects to your body.

A lack of sunlight in the winter leads to what's known as "winter blues" or Seasonal Affective Disorder (SAD), a mood disorder associated with depressive episodes and depression-related fatigue. SAD occurs in some people during fall and winter due to a melatonin imbalance caused by the lack of exposure to sunlight in the short days of those seasons. SAD's depressive symptoms are typically more pronounced between January and February. It's also believed that SAD is due in part to light deprivation that can negatively affect mood.

Like all other maladies, a good diet with regular exercise is essential if you have symptoms of SAD. You also should increase your light exposure by opening drapes, using brighter light bulbs, taking walks outdoors on sunny days during the winter months, and cranking up the light inside when it's dark and gray outside. You also can use light therapy by use of a special light box to treat SAD.

The Least You Need to Know

◆ Stress is caused by anything that provokes your body's systems to react with a physical and, over time, damaging stress response. Stressors include injury; illness; weddings, moving, and career advancement.

◆ Chronic fatigue is often the result of the stress on your body caused by the cumulative effect of fatigue stressors, including poor diet; unhealthy behaviors, illness, and environmental toxins.

◆ Stress-reduction techniques include slow deep breathing, visualizing health and well-being, stretching, other slow deliberate exercises, yoga, and Tai Chi.

◆ The emotional freedom technique (EFT) is a method of psychological acupressure that can be used each day to deal with negative emotional states and even some illness, including aspects of fatigue.

◆ Prayer and mediation have been used since the beginning of time to restore and maintain a sense of inner peace and to assist in health and healing.

◆ We all need a daily dose of sunlight to produce vitamin D, to prevent many diseases (including depression), and to stay healthy.

Chapter 15

Mood Boost

In This Chapter

- ◆ Stay positive to stay healthy
- ◆ Everyone needs support
- ◆ Accept and forgive for healing
- ◆ Alleviating boredom and loneliness
- ◆ The power of journaling
- ◆ Don't forget to have fun

Remember the Nat King Cole song "Smile"?

> "Smile though your heart is aching, smile even though it's breaking. When there are clouds in the sky, you'll get by if you smile through your fear and sorrow …"

Chances are that song has put a tear in your eye at least once. And maybe it's because on some level you know that there is some truth to Nat's bittersweet prescription to smile. While pretending to be happy is not an antidote to conditions like depression, actually working on being happy, positive, upbeat, and self-confident are going to help give you energy, boost your immune function, and actually help decrease your risk of high blood pressure, heart disease, stroke, and cancer. It's thought that negativity is a possible cause of fatigue, possibly because being negative contributes to stress, and by now you know that fatigue is one of your body's signals of something wrong.

If you are going to fight your fatigue, smiling, staying positive, finding ways to boost your mood, and having regular fun will help tremendously. There are many ways to keep positive, and this chapter looks at just a few.

Laughter and Why You Need to Stay Positive

Positive thinking, laughter's closest cousin, is another force to be reckoned with. Positive thinking saturates the brain with words and imagery that are advantageous to growing, expanding, and succeeding. When you are continually positive, you expect and receive a level of success no matter what the outcome. A positive person will take seemingly negative situations and flip them into positives, thus moving forward. Laughter and overall positivity are in fact self-care methods to deal with anxiety, stress, and depression.

How many times have you watched a comedy that has left you laughing or spent time with friends talking and laughing? It left you feeling good, right?

There are interesting and compelling studies being conducted by cardiologists at the University of Maryland Medical Center in Baltimore indicating that laughter might help prevent heart disease. These studies indicate that people with heart disease tend to react to everyday life less positively. They laugh less, are angrier, and more hostile than people without heart disease even with the positive situations in their lives.

In The Know

"The old saying that 'laughter is the best medicine,' definitely appears to be true when it comes to protecting your heart. We don't know yet why laughing protects the heart, but we know that mental stress is associated with impairment of the endothelium, the protective barrier lining our blood vessels. This can cause a series of inflammatory reactions that lead to fat and cholesterol build-up in the coronary arteries and ultimately to a heart attack."

—Michael Miller, M.D., F.A.C.C., Laughter and the heart researcher, director of the Center for Preventive Cardiology at the University of Maryland Medical Center.

This research is beginning to confirm that laughter and the simple act of smiling offer some of the same health benefits as a mild workout, including increased heart rate, vasodilatation of the blood vessels, increasing the level of infection-fighting antibodies, boosting the levels of immune cells, lowering blood sugar levels, promoting relaxation and sleep, suppressing levels of stress hormones like epinephrine, and even relieving pain by boosting levels of endorphins.

Although researchers are just starting to look at the power of laughter and being positive, spiritual leaders, some physicians, nearly all comedians, and our moms and grandmas have always known that laughing simply depowers unfortunate life situations such as illness. Today, even hospitals are prescribing mirthful laughter with humor programs that include clowns, comedy carts with costumes and funny props, and humor rooms with comedy television channels.

Humor can make events less overwhelming while deflecting anger, tension, and frustration. Laughing at oneself without self-degradation actually can boost your self-esteem and self-acceptance while increasing your ability to connect with and accept other people.

Humor produces energy. We end up making more eye contact, touching others more, and becoming more active, possibly doing the work we need to accomplish a necessary task.

Humor helps us replace distressing emotions with pleasurable feelings. Try laughing and feeling anger, depression, anxiety, guilt, or bitterness at the same time. It's hard to do. And by laughing with others, we have a sense of camaraderie, a "we're in this together" mentality.

Weeding Out the Negative

Researchers have known for quite some time that happier people tend to be in better health than those that are negative. And current findings such as a recent study published in the *American Journal of Epidemiology* indicate that happiness and other positive emotions are associated with favorable health and biological responses that are protective to your health. The study, "Neuroendocrine and Inflammatory Factors Associated with Positive Affect in Healthy Men and Women," found that men and women with happier moods had lower average cortisol levels even when factors such as age, weight, smoking, and income are considered.

So how do you get happy and stay positive? Let's first look at typical characteristics of positive people who seem to operate differently than negative people. The positive person tends to see and expect great things to happen in her life. She exudes happiness and goodwill and success in her body language. She attracts other people because, just like laughter, a positive attitude creates a sense of energy, a twinkle in the eyes, and an aura of happiness.

Because both positive and negative thinking are contagious, positive people tend to gravitate to other positive people and avoid those who are giving out negativity. Negativity is as contagious as the common cold. But, unlike a cold, it sometimes never goes away. It's also a somewhat inherited condition passed down through generations of pessimistic whiners.

But not to worry—there is a cure! First, notice how much you complain and instead replace your whine with something positive. If you don't think that will work and feel that you need to continually belabor all your problems, consider a few things. Has complaining or worrying ever done anything to solve your problems? Has it moved you forward into a better situation? Has complaining brought you new friends, helped you to make more money, or brought you closer to any success? No, and that defeating attitude not only causes you failure, but also damages your immune system causing you to feel as bad physically as you do mentally.

In 2006 Will Bowen, a Missouri minister, suggested that his congregation use purple bracelets to examine their success at doing away with complaining from their lives. His campaign was such a success that he began a website www.acomplaintfreeworld. org, which has sent close to 5 million purple Complaint Free bracelets to people in over 80 countries.

In The Know

"Your thoughts create your world and your words indicate your thoughts. When you eliminate complaining from your life you will enjoy happier relationships, better health and greater prosperity. This simple program helps you set a trap for your own negativity and redirect your mind towards a more positive and rewarding life."

—*Will Bowen is the Lead Minister at Christ Church Unity in Kansas City, Missouri and creator of "A Complaint Free World."*

Instead of telling yourself how bad things are and creating self-fulfilling prophecies, visualize your situations as favorable while using positive words in your mind and conversation. Smile whenever you can, even at strangers. When you look up from getting something out of your purse or wallet with a smile and catch a stranger's eye, it makes BOTH of you feel good.

Banish negative thoughts and replace them with positive ones. You might find this ridiculously hard to do at first, but after a while you can retrain your mind to focus on good and ignore bad. If you have deeply ingrained negative thinking, emotional freedom techniques (EFTs), as described in Chapter 15, can be an effective tool to help you to think more positively. Eventually, you're going to find you actually are one of those people who has a good attitude and is attracting good people and things into your life.

Whatever your circumstances are at the present moment, expect and verbalize favorable results in regard to your finances, health, relationships, and other situations and acknowledge forward momentum and improvement no matter how miniscule. Given time, your circumstances are likely to change for the better. Changing your attitude can shift the focus of the meaning and power you put on situations. Something that at one time you belabored as catastrophic can end up being just a tolerable annoyance— or it might go away completely.

People who use the sort of negating language such as *always* and *never* are going to continue always never getting what they want except their desire to disrupt your life and dreams. Negative people in your life also have the effect of being counter-supportive or toxic, and the head games they create might be continually sucking vital energy from you. If you are dealing with feelings of inadequacy or any type of low self-esteem, the last thing you need are critical, negative people in your life.

 Energy Bar

Evict any people from your life, even family members, who are continually putting you down. It wastes energy and causes an increase in negative energy (bad vibes, head games) to be involved with someone on any level who is not "on your side."

Learn how to not react to people who seem to set you up for arguments or to suck you into their negative conversations. It takes much less energy to make a neutral comment like "oh really" than it is to try to debate with a complainer or an expert at contradiction. In essence, deflect any sort of energy drains by not getting sucked into them.

One of the most prevalent and somewhat accepted forms of negativity is gossip (when defined as "personal or intimate rumors or facts, especially when malicious," as is often the underlying intention). While there's a lot of interest in the pros and cons of gossip for the purpose of reducing negativity in your life, looking at your "malicious gossip quotient" just might be in order. Malicious gossip is hard to resist because it can be deliciously enticing and entertaining for the moment and gives you a fleeting, albeit false, sense of power. But the reality is that this sort of gossip causes you to lose trust and credibility and makes you mistrust others and worry about what others are saying about you. Gossip creates internal and external conflict (negativity) and decreases the morale of everyone involved. It undercuts your efforts at staying positive, pure and simple.

Just like changing your internal dialogue, changing what you say about others creates positive vibes about you at the same time it lifts the morale and confidence of yourself and others. Not gossiping is empowering! If you feel that urge to gossip, try turning the conversation into praising another person; you might be surprised at how you will gain a little more positive power along with heaps of integrity and trust.

How to Get the Support You Need

"No man is an island" is a well-known quote from John Donne (1572–1631) meaning that human beings don't flourish when isolated from others. And aside from just the company of others, we all need our feelings to be validated and to be encouraged, praised, and comforted. In other words, we need our own personal cheerleading section for positive feedback, to get us over hurdles, and to help propel us continually forward. We need a shoulder to cry on and someone to make us laugh, to listen to us vent, and to offer advice.

Many people turn to their families, friends, or significant others for support. But sometimes circumstances are such that your friends and loved ones don't understand or can't understand what you are going through. Some things also might be too much of a strain on relationships, and at those times you might need an outside source of support.

The first step in getting support is to somehow ask for it or seek it out. In today's world, there are support groups in online forums for just about any situation, illness, or circumstance. Because of the Internet, you might find someone half a world away to connect with for support and friendship. If you can't find the atmosphere you are looking for in existing forums, you can easily start one yourself even with very little computer tech savvy. See Appendix C for a list of support groups and message boards you can start out with. As you gain Internet experience, you will find there are many different support groups and online forums to choose from.

Another critical component in getting support is to be a part of something. Join a church, club, or support group, or offer to volunteer. Being forthright and honest in your quest for a support group or person can help lead you in the right direction. You might hook up with the right person just by talking about your needs to someone else, including your doctor. You might be able to find an affordable therapist, a social worker, a school counselor, or even a church volunteer to lend an ear. It doesn't matter if you find a formal support group; connect with someone over the Internet; or find a therapist, spiritual guide, or counselor. What matters is that a little support can help make a vast difference in your healing process. A word of caution, be very careful in meeting people online. People are very often not who they present themselves to be in chat rooms and message boards. Never give personal details about yourself and use caution when you arrange to meet an Internet friend in person. Pick a public place and make sure that a friend or family member knows your plans.

Acceptance, Understanding, and Forgiving

If you have ever listened to the eulogy of a person who has died a peaceful death after a long illness, chances are you heard that he celebrated and enjoyed life. Many people who face a terminal illness have epiphanies about accepting their lot so that they can use the time they have left to fulfill other more beneficial purposes, including attaining inner peace and happiness. Because they accept that their time is limited, they choose to use it in the most productive and fulfilling way they possibly can.

No matter where you are in life, acceptance of yourself and circumstances gives you the peace of mind to use your energy to focus on healthy behaviors. You can begin to overcome anything you previously considered a weakness by accepting yourself and your life on its terms. By resisting each urge to self-denigrate, to belabor your problems, your illness, and your lot in life, you begin to have more power over them and your courage will blossom.

 Slip-Ups

Negativity is nonproductive and energy draining. Focusing on the negative in thoughts and in words only causes it to grow, get bigger, and become more all-consuming.

Acceptance has to be partnered with forgiving yourself and others. Unforgiveness is a poisonous prison and sometimes is so deeply rooted that it takes some time and effort to accomplish. Even if you feel you can't forgive yourself or someone else, begin simply by verbalizing your desire to forgive. The more you do this, the more you will actually instill that desire in your heart so you can reach a place where you do feel forgiving.

Researchers have studied behaviors such as holding on to grudges, anger, and bitterness and correlated these behaviors with long-term health problems such as hypertension and stroke. Forgiveness, on the other hand they've seen, offers numerous benefits, including:

- Lower blood pressure and heart rate

- Stress reduction

- Less hostility and improved anger management skills

- Lower risk of alcohol or substance abuse

- Fewer depression and anxiety symptoms

- Chronic pain reduction

- More friendships and healthier relationships

- Improved religious or spiritual well-being

- Improved emotional and mental well-being

Dealing with Boredom and Loneliness

Boredom and fatigue can both be indirect consequences of fatigue. Depending on your level of fatigue, you might be in a place of loss either temporarily or permanently. You might have lost your job, your career goals, or even your identity on some level. Due to rearranged priorities, your focus might now be shifted causing you to feel disconnected from what might have been your routine into uncharted territory and leaving you to carve out a new direction. You might need some time to rethink your priorities and establish healthier behaviors. You might not fit into the mold of what your friends are doing now. You might have had to slow down and say no to activities you've identified as unhealthy. You might find yourself lonely and bored.

You can make getting healthier your job focus. Taking the following steps can help you to feel fulfilled, reconnect with yourself, and perhaps form additional relationships:

◆ Schedule some regular walks and purposefully stopping to notice some interesting things, plants, yards, rocks, shops, or people along the way.

◆ Take the time to relax. Read a good book. Listen to some relaxing music. Go to your local bookstore and hang out while browsing different sections; you might even meet others with your same interests.

◆ Look for community activities or groups to join such as a cooking, fitness, nutrition, or health group.

◆ Start a support group in your home to get you connected to others to help you work together toward your common goal of winning your fight against fatigue.

◆ Look in the newspaper for interesting events and functions you can attend; you might meet someone there.

◆ Ask friends over for a meal or to watch a movie.

◆ Volunteer at a hospital, an animal shelter, a school, or some other organization. Paying it forward can help you to feel connected to others and more fulfilled.

◆ Write letters and emails to servicemen and women overseas.

◆ Go to church and join a church group. Even if you feel very ill, you can still volunteer to do something low-key such as making phone calls for a church ministry.

◆ Engage in politics and current events such as health and illness issues by writing letters to magazines, leaving comments on online blogs, or writing to your congressperson.

Journaling Your Recovery

Chronicling your journey of healing is a great way to identify progress thereby motivating yourself to continue and even to step up your efforts. By looking back over time and seeing how far you've come, you can stop any feelings of defeat or frustration that might be trying to rear their ugly heads.

Your journal can include your plan for recovery including all the aspects outlined in this book, such as your treatment plan including such things as diet, exercise, medications, supplements, and stress reduction. Your recovery is much more evident when you see it illustrated over time. Instead of not thinking about the future, simply free-falling, and taking things as they come, you can use your physical, mental, and emotional power or the mind-body connection to influence your healing process.

You can use the written word by journaling to write letters of forgiveness to yourself and others to validate your feelings, release unhealthy emotions, and let them go.

Writing a *blog* can connect you with others who are going through the same experiences. It can foster a new sense of camaraderie and creativity. Blogs give you the opportunity to give and receive advice and support from others while chronicling your journey.

def•i•ni•tion

Blogs are online diaries (Web-logs) that are easy, are free to set up, and have the added advantage of being able to both give and receive support along the way. By writing a blog, you can connect with people for support, friendship, and validation all around the world.

Whatever you use to record your thoughts, a journal is a time-tested method to foster healing, creativity, and change. You don't have to keep your blog or journal forever; it might be a temporary but useful prescription you can delete or discard after it has fulfilled its purpose. Or who knows, it might end up as a bestseller or feature film someday. Your life is a fascinating journey no matter who you are, where you are, what life has handed you, or what you are doing in your life.

Are You Having Fun Yet?

"All work and no play makes Jack a dull boy" is an expression handed down through time that might have begun with the Egyptian sage Ptahhoptep (2400 B.C.E.) who wrote, "One that reckoneth accounts all the day passeth not a happy moment." In other words, if you never take time off from work you end up boring, bored, and possibly sick and fatigued. Mind-body health requires a balance of work, play, and rest—to be healthy and heal, you need to include regular fun in your life.

Schedule daily fun. Fun doesn't have to be expensive or even take a lot of time; it's simply anything you find pleasurable in your life. For example, if you love flowers, plan on buying some flowers when you shop for food and spend some time each week making a beautiful arrangement to enjoy.

Create an environment of fun and relaxation both at home and at work. You can liven up your work surroundings or your desk by thinking of creative ways to continually redesign your space. For example, bring in a small chalk board to write funny and/or inspirational phrases that will make you and your co-workers laugh.

The point is that having fun is good for you and enjoying your life affects your health in positive ways. Everyone has different ideas of what is fun, but if you are working too much and putting fun on the sidelines, it's time to schedule in some regular fun.

Importance of Me Time

If you think that your kids, your spouse, or your work can't live without you and therefore are putting all your energy into them and none into yourself, you are going to lose yourself. You might reach a point where your kids grow up and don't really need you as much anymore, you might lose your job or retire, or your relationships might go south, and you will be too sick, too burned-out, or too overwhelmed to function. Then what will happen?

In The Know
"We wouldn't feel good if the people we loved didn't have Me Time. What we want for others we should also want for ourselves."
—*Pepper Schwartz, Ph.D., author, speaker, and professor of sociology at the University of Washington, Seattle*

Nurturing yourself is an integral part of physical and emotional health and healing. If you have been spread too thin, you might have forgotten how to nurture yourself or you may just never have known how. Along with all the other responsibilities in your busy life, taking care and caring for yourself should be one of your priorities.

Pampering Yourself

A little pampering helps you to relax and gives you time to reflect on things other than stressful responsibilities. Me Time also helps to remind you of the importance of you, and it helps illustrate your importance to others which in turn works to lift your self-esteem and your image to others.

Take a short break between life's realities with a massage or facial or in a hot tub so you can return de-stressed, refreshed, and relaxed to your responsibilities. Spending some alone time relaxing allows you the opportunity for a little meditation, self-reflection, and creative problem-solving.

Giving yourself Me Time can actually create a sense of having more time because you will be less frazzled, feel more in control and more satisfied, and be able to take care of your responsibilities more efficiently.

Vacations

Vacations give you a time to recharge, increase creativity, and prevent burnout. Regular vacations keep you healthy because getting away can decrease or eliminate stress, making you stronger and more able to deal with your work and life when you return.

More than 12,000 men were followed for nine years in a study called Multiple Risk Factor Intervention Trial; the results were published in a 2000 issue of *Journal of Psychosomatic Medicine*. Men who vacationed were found to be healthier and lived longer than those who didn't. Studies that have focused on women show that women who vacation experience less depression and anxiety, a better quality of life, and better performance at work.

Many people simply forget to plan for vacations. And others have an all-or-nothing attitude. But you don't need to book a flight and stay in a hotel out of state or abroad to experience a vacation. Rather you can plan getaways that include day road trips, local walks or hikes, wine tasting, overnight camping, or any other activity you enjoy.

Personal Interests and Hobbies

Fulfilling relationships, work, and your time off all have a positive impact on your sense of satisfaction in life, your health, and your well-being. The more contentment or substance you have in your life, the more well-rounded and satisfied you are likely to be.

Of course, any physically active leisure hobbies are going to give you positive health benefits: keeping excess weight off, keeping your cardiovascular system fit, keeping your bones healthy, and giving you a sense of well-being. Sports activities also are ways to become involved and have fun with others, meet new people, and otherwise socialize.

Hobbies and other personal interests have other benefits, too. For example, keeping your mind active by playing cards or board games, solving crossword puzzles, or learning a musical instrument or language is now being shown in studies to help prevent Alzheimer's disease and other types of dementia. Your brain is a muscle that seems to atrophy if it's not exercised.

Energy Bar

Going for a solitary walk, bike ride, or swim can give you time to think, quietly problem-solve, pray, meditate, or otherwise recharge.

When you have personal interests and hobbies in your life, you tend to stay more connected to others, you might be less lonely and have more social interactions, you have more activities to exercise your brain, and you are able to transition from different seasons of life such as work to retirement more easily. Hobbies don't have to cost anything either. You can start walking and bird watching or rock collecting with just the cost of some good walking shoes. If you want to walk with others, you can join events that walk for causes. Just using your brain to think about activities to join that you will enjoy gives you the benefit of exercising your brain!

The Least You Need to Know

◆ Smiling, laughing, having a positive attitude, and having regular fun are associated with health benefits including a longer and happier life.

◆ Negativity in your attitude and in those around you is a toxic poison. You can banish negative thoughts and behaviors and evict negative people from your life, thereby creating healthy favorable self-fulfilling prophesies.

◆ Seek out and ask for support so that you get the validation, encouragement, and advice you need to get healthy and move forward.

◆ Accepting where you are today and your circumstances, while forgiving yourself and others, gives you an edge for healing. Bitterness and unforgiveness are both toxic prisons that will poison all your other efforts to heal.

◆ By journaling, you can keep track of your progress and become more motivated to make beneficial changes in your life. Journals can be written on paper, online in *blogs*, or in a word processing program on your computer.

◆ Don't forget to have fun! It's essential to decompress, to exercise your mind, to expand your horizons, and to escape the daily grind of life.

Chapter 16

Winning the Fight Against Fatigue

In This Chapter

◆ Adding up your fatigue stressors

◆ Understanding the effects of triggers

◆ Listening to cues

◆ Creating your personal plan

◆ Doing the work, giving it time, and believing!

This book isn't about managing your symptoms or a manual about how to be a professional patient. It's about becoming healthy and, dare I say, cured. It all really boils down to "person heal thyself." By now, you have had a chance to pinpoint the many areas of your life that are stressed and have added up to an enormous load you are carrying. Whatever challenges you have in front of you, I hope that you are pumped because you can do it!

This chapter helps you put it all together so you can start moving forward. So, put any thoughts of being a victim aside and begin to think of being victorious instead. The great thing about this program of improved habits and decreased stressors is that it's all an incredible lifestyle that is going to put you on the fast track to living a long and healthy life.

So roll up your sleeves and get ready!

Adding Up Your Stressors

If you have been taking notes all along, then you might already have a list of your stressors. If not, you can use the following fatigue stressor checklist to get a good view of the cumulative amount of fatigue stressors you have. Go through each category and put a check next to each stressor that applies to you. In the "other" category, list any additional stressors you feel apply.

Physiological

Low blood sugar___ Infections___ Diseases___ Illness___ Surgery___ Allergies___
Chemical Sensitivity___ Obesity___
Menopause___
Other (list) _____

_____

Emotional

Depression___ Anxiety___ Anger and Rage___
Emotional Trauma___ Eating Disorder___
Extreme Stress___ Negativity___
Other (list) _____

_____

Environmental

Personal Care and Household Toxins___ Pollution___ Mercury___

Brain Poisons (MSG, Food Additives, Chemical/Artificial Sugars)_____

_____

Other (list) _____

_____

Lifestyle

Diet (Junk, Processed, or Restaurant Food)___ Addictions___ Workaholism ___
Lack of Conditioning___ Overexercise___
Overeating___ Undereating___ Perfectionism___ Chronic Dehydration___
Coffee___ Stimulants___
Other (list) _____

_____

Issues with Sleep and Rest

Shift Work___ Frequent Travel___ Insomnia___
Sleep Disorders___ Sleep Debt___
Sleep Deprivation___
Other (list) _____

_____

Current and Past Medical Treatments

Chemotherapy___ Radiation___
Overuse of Prescription and OTC Medication_____
Other (list) _____

_____

Support Issues

Lack of Support___ Feeling Unappreciated___ Abuse___ Burnout___ Toxic
Relationships___
Other (list) _____

_____

Miscellaneous Stressors

Lack of Friends___ Inability to Relax or Have Fun___ No Social Outlets___ No
Hobbies___ Lacking Content in Life___
Other (list) _____

_____

If you have infections, diseases, or illnesses contributing to your fatigue, you
need to address them as your doctor recommends. But also be aware that even
with a chronic illness, you can live a healthier life by improving your lifestyle
habits and behaviors. You can even turn it around by improving your lifestyle
habits and behaviors.

Slip-Ups

Don't feel you have no control over your life, even if you have severe fatigue or Chronic Fatigue Syndrome (CFS). You have a great deal of control through the decisions you make everyday. You make choices everyday that have a positive or negative impact on your health.

Although no one stressor is more important than the next, there are certain "biggies" that need to be on the top of your list for change. They are requisite for the healing process to begin.

First and foremost, you need to start getting the sleep that you need for good health. Second, you need to eat a good breakfast of real whole food followed by a lunch and a dinner of real food, along with healthy snacks. Third, you need to get some exercise. If you are doing these three things, then you should begin to see some improvement in a very short time.

Eliminating sugar and caffeine are other relatively easy fixes for most people. Don't forget that sugar is a primary component in processed food! But first, you need to cut out the more obvious sources like that donut and coffee you "use" to boost your energy. Remember, they actually are stealing from you in the long run. When fatigue is robbing you of your life, you won't feel these changes are really deprivation, but rather a trade-off for excellent health.

Other stressors might be more difficult to deal with or eliminate. The best approach is to figure out what you can easily do first and then, when you gain more energy, you will find that the other changes are less challenging. And it's not all about eliminating stressors—it's also about enjoying the things you are supposed to enjoy, including your meals, your entertainment, your exercise, and your rest and relaxation. Give yourself permission to start enjoying your life.

Identifying Triggers

Over time, you might have figured out some of the activities or events that trigger your fatigue. You understand that it means you also must avoid and minimize those triggers. Keeping a diary or allocating a portion of your journal to track your triggers might help you to steer clear of making the same self-defeating mistakes.

One of the most obvious triggers is overdoing activities that cause you to have post exertional fatigue. But overdoing can be understated, and that is when understanding certain subtleties can help. In some people, overdoing it can involve something as seemingly benign as talking or loud and animated conversation. Even stimulants like loud music or emotionally charged events can result in fatigue. Other people might not tolerate alcohol or caffeine in any amount, hot weather, cold and damp weather, certain medications or food, or being the slightest bit dehydrated. It goes without saying that sleep deprivation, drinking too much, eating junk and processed food, smoking, working out when tired, over- or undereating, and all other fatigue stressors outlined in this book are obvious triggers.

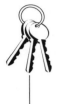

Energy Bar _____

Keeping your blood sugar level is doable, but it usually means planning ahead. If you are going out to run errands, plan on packing a snack or even a lunch to take with you. In fact, regular planning for meals ahead of time removes the trigger of low blood sugar and takes it permanently out of the equation.

Ignoring triggers isn't going to get you anywhere. If you are made ill by perfume, then you have to take steps to not be around it. If that means talking to someone about it or moving your workspace, you need to do that. The good news about chemical sensitivity is that you can overcome it somewhat by improving your immune function, but you won't be able to do that if you continue to stay in a perfumed or toxic environment.

Emotional stress often triggers fatigue. The source often comes from feelings of defeat and beating yourself up. Or it might stem from believing that others don't understand your plight. So tell yourself you are doing the best you can do and stop the negative inner dialogue. In the case of other people, briefly explain you have fatigue and how it differs from being tired or exhausted. Give them a short rundown on your limitations and how you are dealing with them. Then let it go. Some people will understand and others won't, but don't internalize this by making it your problem.

Listening to Your Body

Chances are you don't remember how fatigue crept into your life, but removing it and keeping it gone is going to take respecting and listening to the cues your body is giving you. You have the greatest internal monitor for up-to-date and accurate reports of minute-to-minute changes and cues that are taking place within your own body. If you actually listen and heed your body's own warning system, you'll find you know a lot more about what is making you sick and how to channel that information into wellness.

Many of us take our cues from other people instead of ourselves. But, just because others are inflicting self-harm doesn't mean that you should also. In fact, those people who are wearing their self-abuse as a badge of honor are likely to approach you at some point in the future for advice on how you manage to function so well and never become sick. This is because self-abuse can go on only for so long, and those coffee guzzlers who burn the midnight oil and neglect their self-care are going to succumb at some point to fatigue or some other health condition.

Developing the important self-help tool of listening to your body first requires that you understand what is normal for you, what your personal limitations are, and what you can and cannot tolerate. What is normal for you can take the form of knowing, for example, that you can't eat that piece of lasagna at a late-night supper, have cheesecake and coffee for desert, smoke a few cigarettes or a cigar with a nightcap, and then go to sleep effortlessly and sleep soundly. Instead, if you engage in that sort of destructive behavior, you are likely to feel hammered when you wake up—if you can get to sleep at all. And although some people can do that or engage in any other version of self-neglect and abuse, are they really a picture of health?

In The Know

"Unless you learn to notice and be bothered by the early, subtle stages of illness, you will lose your chances of managing your body through its changing cycles by simple means and will find yourself more and more dependent on outside practitioners and the costly interventions of modern hospital medicine."

—Andrew Weil, M.D., Spontaneous Healing

It is important to know what is normal for your own body. Although most people are in tune with the symptoms of illness that they perceive as radical changes in their bodies and are quick to see their doctor, they often ignore minor signals that slowly can lead to serious illness. On the other hand, people engaged in self-abuse often end up ignoring the rather obvious warning signs, which typically is what happens in the majority of fatigue cases.

The remedy involves listening to your body to find out how you got to the point of fatigue. Many cues seem straightforward—for example, hunger should signal eating, but the reality is that not everyone responds in a healthy way to cues. So signals that should lead to normal behaviors like eating are interrupted and replaced with fatigue stressors such as downing coffee or eating sugary snacks. You then get a cue that feels like a headache and instead of realizing that your blood sugar has been on a roller-coaster ride, you take an over-the-counter (OTC) pain reliever and down a diet soda.

By not listening to begin with, you end up numb to the real cues and you medicate the symptoms that follow with bad behaviors.

Another typical scenario follows those who are sedentary but who don't understand that their muscles are becoming rigid and tight, cramping, and spasming due to deconditioning. The typical consequences for a deconditioned person is developing pain or easily getting fatigued, which leads to further avoiding any exercise or activity. The person then ends up fearful of exercise because of his pain and exercise intolerance and then increases his ingestion of pain medication followed by insomnia, sleep deprivation, and depression. Too many people are being medicated for depression because they didn't listen to the first subtle cues. You might not even realize that your muscles are talking to you!

You can fine-tune your listening ability if you stop abusing your body (this term may be a little judgmental) and begin to open yourself up to the finer nuances of your body. Think about it the next time you get a headache or stomachache. Can you connect that distress with something fixable in your behavior or lifestyle? Try writing down all your subtle cues along with the obvious symptoms and distresses in your journal so you can make the connections you need to and correct the offending behaviors.

Aside from documenting symptoms and cues, you can hear your body loud and clear by measuring your waist, weight, blood pressure, and (if you feel ill) your temperature. While you are changing your eating habits, it's also a good time to measure those other objective signs so you can get even more motivated when you see such progress as achieving a normal blood pressure and a decrease in your weight and waist measurement.

> **In The Know**
>
> Normal blood pressure is 120/80 or lower; 140/90 or higher is considered high blood pressure. Prehypertension is between 120 and 139 for the top number and between 80 and 89 for the bottom number.

Your Personal Plan

Depending on the severity of your fatigue, your plan is going to vary, but the basic protocol needs to look something like the following:

◆ Make an appointment with your doctor for necessary tests to rule out the common medical causes of fatigue, including anemia, infection, disease, and any sleep disorders.

◆ Get help from therapy, a support group, your church, or an online forum. Make sure that you are part of a group or community whose goal is health and healing and not simply how to manage symptoms or a continuation of any victim role. See Appendix C for Internet support groups and online forums.

◆ Take a serious look at your diet. Making basic changes can help you to ease up on your adrenals and increase your energy while decreasing your cravings for caffeine and sugar. Make plans to overhaul your diet by removing processed food and junk food and incorporating real food into your diet. Remember that eating real food requires planning ahead with grocery lists and meal plans.

◆ Examine your typical behaviors for reacting to stress. If you are using drugs or alcohol, you will find that at least eliminating the nightcap will give you more restorative sleep so that you have the energy to make bigger changes in that area. Using stress-reduction techniques along with methods such as the emotional freedom technique (EFT) will give you the tools you need to succeed.

◆ Consider why you are burning the candle at both ends and what you can do to create more balance in your life. Write out your plan for how you can delegate some of what you think you had to do before, how you can stop and smell the roses every day, and what things you can stop doing that aren't really necessary at all.

◆ Get your bedtime ritual going with a plan for instituting healthy sleeping habits and sleep hygiene.

◆ Be alert to any possible food sensitivities you might have that may be adding to your fatigue. Cleaning up your diet and eliminating some of the chronic offenders, including additives in food, will help you heal your GI track.

◆ Stay hydrated throughout the day by drinking about one half of your body weight in ounces of pure, clean water every day.

◆ Find a source for good quality supplements, including a multivitamin, cod liver oil, calcium and magnesium combination, probiotics, and others that you might need to support your immune function.

◆ Get some exercise everyday so you can relieve stress and depression and sleep better while getting in shape. Make a realistic plan so you will stick with it. Planning on doing five minutes of yoga four or five times a week might be more realistic than planning to work out sixty minutes three times a week. People with severe fatigue need to follow graded exercise recommendations.

◆ Get rid of environmental toxins in your home for personal and household tasks. Find a source for chemical-free personal care and household products. This measure is one of the easiest changes you can make.

◆ Incorporate some simple fatigue-reducing measures into your life such as doing some deep breathing throughout the day, getting outside and getting some sun every day, getting up from your desk and stretching and walking around on a regular basis (including resting your eyes every hour from the computer), and sitting down at the table to eat and enjoying your food.

◆ Practice forgiveness every day, including forgiving yourself. Clean up the negative in all areas of your life, your thoughts, your relationships, and your behaviors.

◆ Work on bad habits and vices such as smoking, drugs, and excessive drinking. Make your plan to quit and put together the resources you need to make it happen.

So, let's run that down simply: if you get eight hours of sleep every night; take high-quality supplements; exercise; stay hydrated; restore your intestinal flora with probiotics if necessary; and stop all bad habits like smoking, drinking, and using drugs, you are setting the stage for gradual improvement in symptoms. These changes might be more difficult for some than for others, but they are all fundamental in winning your fight and staying fatigue free.

Depending on your level of fatigue and overall state of health, you may begin to see improvement right away in a matter of weeks or longer in some cases. Don't give up if you don't see the improvement you expect right away because it may take longer then you expect. Perhaps setting the stage for slow gradual improvement in symptoms is important here.

Healing Takes Time and Commitment

At the top of your list you need to strike off despair and disbelief and insert hope, belief, and confidence that you can win your fight. Because fatigue can cause you to feel confused and fearful, you might have gotten to a point where you are resigned to living out the rest of your life with this reduced or even nonexistent quality of life that your fatigue has caused.

Recognizing improvements can be frustrating, or you might feel you are not making any improvements at all. The first thing you need to realize is that all the interventions you are instituting are improvements unto themselves. Because fatigue is so subtle, it probably has crept very slowly into your life. Being able to actually acknowledge improvements might take closely examining understated changes that are happening in your health.

If you have serious fatigue like CFS or even severe chronic fatigue, some of the first major improvements you will experience are waking up not feeling fatigued. Because you are so excited about this new development, it might be difficult to continue pacing yourself throughout the day. You can then find yourself relapsing into a bad fatigue state. This is why it's imperative to continue to pace yourself while you are journaling your improvement so you can increase your activity incrementally over time and not jump the gun. The push and pull you experience with severe fatigue caused by overdoing it and suffering post exertional fatigue is defeating. But if you follow the rules outlined for pacing, you can decrease the negative effects that crashing and burning cause.

Energy Bar

Try to find some meaning in what you are going through so you can see the changes as positive and as an avenue for growth. For example, plan on using the benefit of your experience in the future to help others.

The last months (or years of your recovery, depending on the severity of your fatigue) are actually some of the most demanding and downright frustrating. You see doors opening, but you have to enter gradually and obey limitations of staying away from triggers, continuing to say no, and stopping activities before you become tired. It's better to be safe than sorry when it comes to your recovery because it will pay off in the long run. You will find the windows of time when you feel better are getting larger and those when you feel bad are getting smaller.

In most cases, healing fatigue is outside the scope of medicine (only 10 percent have medical causes), so the burden of responsibility is on you. In your healing work, don't forget to take the time you need for such restorative activities as prayer and meditation that are an integral part of reducing pain and healing your nervous system, immune system, adrenal glands, and hormonal system.

Reduce your use of television, news, noise, and other less-obvious stimulants while you increase your time enjoying nature, music, art, good food, reading, and people. Try to foster your creative side by experimenting with new media like drawing, writing, cooking, or even arranging flowers.

It's not uncommon to become fearful of relapse and to avoid altogether those activities you think might bring on more pain and suffering. Understand that as you progress and your times of feeling better increase, your relapses will also be shorter and less harsh. So even though it's good to have a healthy awareness of your limitations, don't let that keep you from moving forward.

On the other hand, be sure to relish and appreciate all your forward momentum. Share your gratitude with others and avoid social isolation at all costs. Nurture your compassionate side and try to spend some time doing things for other people. This will soothe your soul and help give you inner peace.

Your Individual Prognosis

By now you understand that fatigue is a symptom that exists on a continuum from mild to very severe and in some cases can be actual CFS. If you have CFS, you should know that it's a fact that it is one of the most trivialized conditions known to medicine. Very often, you won't get the support, the understanding, or even the validation from friends, families, and doctors that you are as ill as you are. But you don't have to have a diagnosis of CFS to have severe and disabling fatigue. In fact, very few people are actually diagnosed with CFS; however, millions of people are actually disabled with severe and chronic fatigue.

You might have been told that there is no cure for your fatigue and all you can do is to try to manage it. In most cases, this is simply not true. However, it has sprung forth from the premise that there is no medication to cure CFS. That is true, but the reality is that you can heal from CFS if you make the commitment to make the necessary changes in your life. It's a terrible but true irony that the more severe fatigue you have, the harder you have to work to heal from it. The good news is that your healing can happen and your efforts are all going to pay off over time.

Natalie the nurse from previous chapters is a good example of someone who recovered from severe CFS. She first became sick during the time when CFS was not well understood or accepted. Natalie was typical of many people with CFS who went through years of medical tests and misdiagnosis because her doctors didn't understand or know much about CFS. It took nearly five years for Natalie to recover after she eliminated fatigue stressors from her life. If you talk to her now, she would tell you her recovery was not an easy road and that she often felt discouraged and defeated. But she had a strong desire to work toward health and believed her recovery was possible.

No matter if you have severe fatigue like Natalie or you have mild fatigue, you have the benefit of having more knowledgeable doctors in the treatment of fatigue and CFS, years of research studies, acceptance by the medical and general community, more awareness, and the information found in this book.

If you are someone who is waiting for a medical cure to be discovered, try to put that notion aside and focus your energies on the reality that "you" are the cure. There's an interesting observation in medicine that the patients who recover from severe fatigue states such as CFS are the ones who actually believe they will recover. Those who succumb to believing there is no cure while waiting for the magic bullet to appear are the ones who stay sick.

It's also counterproductive to try to figure out a medical reason for your fatigue. If your doctor has run diagnostic tests that have not come up positive for any medical condition and has diagnosed you with CFS or simply told you there is no medical reason, then accept it and move on. People who continue to search for the mysterious disease-producing organism or undiscovered medical condition are only wasting precious time and energy.

In The Know

"People with chronic fatigue syndrome and fibromyalgia can reduce their symptoms and improve their chances of recovery with combined use of mind/body medicine, nutritional medicine, lifestyle and behavior change, and pharmaceutical drugs."

—William Collinge, Ph.D., author of Recovering from the Chronic Fatigue Syndrome: A Guide to Self-Empowerment

---

If you have CFS or Severe Adrenal Fatigue, it might take years for you to recover fully. But during that time you need to be filled with joy and gratitude at the continual improvements you see over time. Every improvement needs to be recognized and appreciated so you can build on your success instead of letting setbacks discourage you and allow any poisonous negativity in. Remember that you are peeling away layer upon layer that has built-up over the years while you are healing the actual cells in your body systems like those in your nervous system and adrenal glands—and all of this takes time.

The timetable to return to good health when you have instituted all the fatigue stressor reduction and elimination measures is at least a month for mild cases of fatigue. It might take you three to six months if you have moderate fatigue. And if your fatigue is very severe, it might take six to nine months to see any improvement, and two or more years for significant improvement to occur. It might then take a couple of years or longer to actually get back to your baseline of the full health you started out with. Your recovery will also depend on the many variables you have, including other diseases and conditions and medical treatment you might be dealing with at the same time.

By now I hope that you see the severity of the impact of stressors and toxins on your health and how you can take the wheel and guide your body and life back to health. Your outcome is in your hands. It's now time to accept the challenge and do the necessary healing work by believing you can heal, refocusing your passion, and channeling it toward a lifestyle that will improve every area of your life, and not only your fatigue.

If you accept doing the work now and make a plan of action that includes making the necessary changes, today is the first day of your improved health and long, healthy, fatigue-free life. Understanding what you need to do and making the decision to change is the first step; the rest is progress. Get excited because tomorrow is a new day and things are definitely going to look better in the morning.

The Least You Need to Know

- You can use the fatigue stressor checklist in this chapter to get a bird's-eye view of the amount of fatigue stressors you have.

- There are certain "biggies" that need to be on the top of your list for change and are requisite for the healing process to begin: getting the sleep you need, eating a good diet, and getting some exercise.

- Figure out what are your triggers causing fatigue such as over doing it, stress, poor diet, and smoking.

- Your plan should involve steps such as seeing your doctor; therapy and/or support groups; a good diet; reducing stress; adequate sleep; staying hydrated; taking high-quality supplements; exercise; quitting bad habits; and getting support from friends or family.

- Mild fatigue can be turned around in about a month; moderate fatigue takes three to six months; and severe fatigue can take six to nine months for some improvement and two years or more for significant life-changing improvement.

- People who heal are those who believe it can happen, do the work, and give it time.

Appendix A

Glossary

acetaminophen   An over-the-counter (OTC) pain reliever.

acquired immune deficiency syndrome or acquired immunodeficiency syndrome (AIDS)   Symptoms and infections that are a result of damage to the immune system.

acupressure   A technique using the fingers to press select points or meridians on the surface of the skin to stimulate the body's natural healing abilities.

acupuncture   A traditional Chinese medicine treatment modality that uses the insertion of very fine needles into defined acupuncture points or meridians on the body where it's believed that energy freely flows during a healthy state.

addiction   The compulsive use of a substance (drugs, alcohol, caffeine, nicotine, even sugar) despite having dangerous, unhealthy, and other negative effects. Addicts have an internal drive to seek the substance primarily to maintain a sense of well-being or comfort.

Addison's disease   Occurs when the adrenal glands produce markedly decreased cortisol, causing fatigue.

adrenal fatigue   A syndrome associated with intense or prolonged stress, indicating the adrenal glands are functioning below the optimal levels.

adrenal glands   The small, triangular-shaped glands located on the top of the kidneys. Their job is to prepare the body for fight-or-flight during times of stress, by releasing "stress" hormones including adrenaline, noradrenaline, and cortisol.

adrenaline   A stress hormone that is activated to increase the heart rate and to elevate blood pressure and energy supplies in the body.

affirmations   A method for improved self-confidence and changing destructive thinking habits by voicing, reading, or writing positive thoughts.

air pollution (smog)   Any abnormal visible or invisible substance found in the air that is a threat to the health of human beings, other life, and the earth itself. It is primarily ozone, carbon monoxide, nitrous oxides, particulate matter, sulfur dioxide, and lead.

allergic reaction   An acquired abnormal inflammatory reaction to a substance (allergen) caused by environmental agents.

allergies   An inflammatory response to substances that aren't actually harmful or the result of immune systems in overdrive from a continual barrage of toxins.

Alpha waves   Brain waves typical of the relaxed state.

alpha lipoic acid   A potent antioxidant that increases production of glutathione in the body helping to dissolve toxins in the liver.

anemia   A below-normal red blood cell count.

anorexia nervosa   A condition in which a person refuses to eat sufficient food to maintain a minimally normal body weight. It sometimes is accompanied by obsessive exercise.

antihistamines   Medications that are used to treat allergic reactions. They also are sedating.

antioxidants   Vitamins and minerals in food that work to remove harmful oxidants or free radicals from the body.

anxiety   An emotional state that includes feeling on edge, tension, fatigue, lack of or low energy, worrying, self-doubt and indecisiveness, difficulty problem-solving, worry about social situations or performance, perfectionism, a tendency to procrastinate, addictive behaviors, depression, trouble controlling emotions or thoughts, and a tendency to be highly sensitive.

art therapists   Skilled professionals who help you unleash your internal imagery on paper, canvas, sculpture, or other art media.